Lymphatic Filariasis

The Quest to Eliminate a 4000-Year-Old Disease

by Malcolm Dean

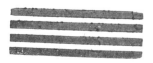

Table of Contents

A Story That Had to Be Chronicled

I was first tipped off that an important international health story was about to break as I was sitting with a panel of health specialists in London judging the annual U.K. community health IMPACT Awards of GlaxoSmithKline (GSK). I was unable to wheedle any more information out of Dr. James Hill, company vice president, during that day. The company was still in confidential talks with the World Health Organization (WHO) about a momentous joint disease elimination programme. Unlike the smallpox and polio campaigns, it would be using drugs. And as its millennium project, GSK was proposing to provide its key drug free of all charges—up to a possible six billion tablets over a 20-year period: the biggest mass drug treatment programme ever.

Launch day itself would have had even more impact but for the fact that the Monica Lewinsky story broke in the U.S. and the Queen Mother had a fall in the U.K. No prizes for guessing which stories dominated the front pages in the respective countries on that day, but the eradication story also received widespread coverage. The launch was in early 1998. Two months later I met Dr. Hill to make a proposal. I was owed 12 weeks of sabbatical leave by my newspaper. I was looking for a worthwhile project. What could be more worthwhile than tracking from the beginning the eradication of a disease? Only one disease, smallpox, had ever been eradicated. The planned eradication of a second was clearly a gripping story. It needed a chronicler. I had only one stipulation. For my reputation—as well as the company's—I had to have

v

complete editorial independence. He was as enthusiastic as I was. Within weeks the commission was agreed.

The report that follows is an account of the last three years as I have watched an inspiring enterprise lift off. Its 20-year goal is intimidating: the elimination of a disease which has 120 million people in its grip and threatens a further 1.2 billion in the 80 poorest countries of the world. Ironically, few have even heard of the disease, lymphatic filariasis (LF), though most will have heard of one condition, elephantiasis. Three years of real momentum has been achieved. An LF Global Alliance comprising the three key international agencies (WHO, the World Bank, UNICEF), multiple numbers of non-government agencies, national aid agencies, leading academic institutions, plus the two drug giants (GSK and Merck & Co., Inc.) has come together to eliminate the disease. It began as an agreement between porcupines without much warmth. But it has grown closer and closer. The first treatments began in 2000: just over three million people in 12 countries. This year (2001), acceleration has begun with a projected 40 million people in 27 countries being treated.

I have met a cast of inspiring people—patients, medics, nurses, community workers, village drug distributors, tropical disease specialists, entomologists, social researchers, earlier eradication team leaders, political leaders, donors, medical historians, and international agency chiefs who have given me hours of their time. I feel privileged to have had the commission.

My first interviews, let alone later ones, with Eric Ottesen, the world's leading LF authority at WHO headquarters in Geneva, and David Addiss, a senior LF researcher at the massive U.S. Centers for Disease Control (CDC) in Atlanta, lasted for over seven hours each. A succession of David's colleagues at CDC—including Pat Lammie and Michael Beach—filled in other huge gaps in my knowledge. Brian Bagnall, director of the GSK's LF programme, suffered a similar series of grillings and astutely guided me to key projects and pilot schemes. He was ably supported by Minne Iwamoto in GSK's Philadelphia office. James Hill even identified the critics of the eradication campaign for me. Dr. G.B.

White, the British entomologist, introduced me to the mosquito world and its 3,500 species.

There are a host of other people, including Carter Center staff in Atlanta (Don Hopkins, Frank Richards, Andy Agle, Craig Withers) and Nigeria (Emmanuel Miri and Abel Eigege—see Chapter Five) who helped expand my education. Dr. Stefanie Meredith of the Mectizan Donation Program gave me my first introduction to river blindness. Bill Foege let me tape him for three hours in the bar of a London hotel. Dr. Gerusa Dreyer in Brazil, Dr. John Gyapong in Ghana and Dr. Kazuyo Ichimori, the WHO co-ordinator in the Pacific were all most hospitable hosts. I was received by all with patience, good humour and a rewarding readiness to inform. A big thank you to all of them—and to various researchers at the London School of Tropical Medicine and the WHO library in Geneva, but particularly to Julie Bettinger at CDC in Atlanta, who cheerfully responded to request after request, in person and by email, for a whole mountain of research studies.

The company has been exemplary. I have had open access and no interference. This is an entirely independent report. The drug industry in 2001 came under heavy media criticism for its pricing and patenting policies on HIV/AIDS drugs. Indeed, I joined in that criticism and my newspaper played a leading role in the media campaign. But these criticisms should not detract from the magnificent efforts of GSK and Merck towards eliminating LF. GSK's offer of free drugs for all LF sufferers until the disease has been eradicated was rightly described by London's Financial Times as "the biggest single act of corporate philanthropy in any industry".

I have been to a succession of schemes round the world, where public health officials were unstinting in their tributes not just to the free drug donations, but the support services they received from the drug companies too. Eric Ottesen, key WHO coordinator of the programme, is equally unequivocal: "GSK deserves far more credit than they have received so far. They have been a selfless partner." Professor Bill Foege, the biggest name in public health, who has played a key role in a succession of control programmes going back four decades—smallpox, polio, river blindness—is unequivocal about the need for public/private alliances if eradication programmes are to succeed (See Chapter One). His International Taskforce on the Eradication of Disease identified six which could be eliminated.

This report is aimed at the non-specialist—including potential donors and funders that are still needed—but I hope there is information here that will be useful for specialists too and future eradication campaigners.

The first chapter includes an overview for busy people—so if they read nothing else, they will have a good grasp of how the campaign came to be launched and the challenge lying ahead. The other chapters follow on naturally. Chapter Two describes the history and pathology of the disease, through the eyes of Sir Patrick Manson, who after discovering the cause of the disease went on to became internationally recognised as the father of tropical medicine just over 100 years ago. Chapter Three reminds people of the living conditions under which LF sufferers live—in Africa, the Caribbean, India, South America and the Pacific—and the community health campaigns being organised to help them. Chapter Four looks in much more detail at the eradication challenge. Chapter Five describes the crucial experiments in Nigeria to run integrated campaigns against two or even three tropical diseases. Chapter Six describes what can be done for existing patients and the inspiring clinics that have been developed by a pioneering doctor in Brazil. The final chapter sets out how a global alliance is built—the key to eradicating a disease.

Happy reading—and don't forget the need for more donors.

CHAPTER ONE

Overview:
The Global Challenge

I t is one of the oldest and most debilitating diseases in the world. The statue of a Pharaoh, created 4,000 years ago, shows clear visible signs of the disease. It is mentioned in the ancient medical texts of China, India, and Persia. The National Museum of Japan has wood-block illustrations, made 1,200 years ago, of the gross disfigurement generated by the disease. It remains today the second leading cause of permanent and long-term disability. Yet few people know its name—lymphatic filariasis—and even fewer know how to pronounce it. This writer had to struggle and understands why the endemic communities produced pithier titles: Big Leg, Big Foot or Gross Foot. Even so, most people are familiar with one of its worst outcomes: elephantiasis, the grossly disfiguring swelling of patients' limbs.

This is the story of an amazingly bold medical gamble: a grand global alliance, involving the biggest players in international health and many of smaller parties too, who have set out to eliminate the disease within 20 years. It is a fascinating and still developing tale. In the history of man, only one disease has ever been eradicated: smallpox, in 1977. If successful, the new campaign will be the first to eliminate a disease by drugs, with the largest mass drug administration programme ever. It is in line to become the second, if the Guinea Worm eradication campaign succeeds, to eliminate a vector borne disease—diseases transmitted by blood sucking insects—and the fourth, after smallpox, polio and Guinea Worm, to be eradicated. There is already a large cast of heroes and heroines (See later chapters), but at the heart of the campaign is an even more inspiring group of people: the patients.

Individuals tend to get submerged by numbers. They shouldn't be—and won't be—but here in a paragraph is the scale by numbers of the daunting challenge the LF Global Alliance faces: over 120 million people in 80 countries suffer from the disease and 1.2 billion—one fifth of the world's population—are at risk. About 44 million suffer from recurrent infections and abnormalities of their renal functions; another 76 million have pre-clinical, internal damage to their lymphatic and renal systems; 10 per cent develop elephantiasis, including massive skin folds, fissures and a weeping cauliflower surface that emits a terrible odour; 15 per cent develop lymphoedema, the swelling of arms, legs and breasts; and 25 million men have developed the least well-known but worst outcome of the disease: hydrocoele, under which the scrotum fills with fluid and swells in extreme cases to the size of footballs or even larger. Corrective surgery is available, but the $30 cost is equivalent to a month's salary in Ghana, or three months' pay in India.

The patients I've met—in Africa, the Caribbean, South America, India and the Pacific Islands—are inspiring for their dignified stoicism. Many have suffered grievously: shame, stigma and sometimes extreme social exclusion but there was little self-pity or complaining. Health workers explained there was another group, too depressed to meet outsiders, who were suicidal and in urgent need of emotional and psychological support. Some societies blame the victims, believing the disease only infects people who have committed a serious sin or community offence: hydrocoele, for example, for adultery. Other societies have been more sympathetic but until recently have been unable to offer any effective treatment for those with the disease.

The psychological consequences of the disease can be disastrous. Patients lose their jobs, suffer serious sexual dysfunction, forfeit their chance of marriage or face divorce because of their disfiguring disease. Even the lucky ones who have found a treatment clinic, have a hard time. Kesnel Guerrier, a young wiry Haitian farmer with a small plot high in the mountains above Leogane, had a four hour journey to the island's only clinic (by foot and overcrowded "tap tap" buses) and four hours back. But he wasn't complaining. Some patients had a two day journey. He was grateful for the new techniques he was learning to control the swellings. His productivity on the farm, already reduced by his chronic conditions, suffered even further losses by acute attacks—fever, chills, nausea, vomiting—that last for about five days. In Ghana and Nigeria, the peasant farmers carried an additional burden, with many acute attacks coinciding with the rainy season, the most active time of the year for farmers. I met fishermen on the Pacific islands of Vanuatu and French Polynesia, where successful eradication campaigns have been launched, who had had to give up their fishing boats because their hydrocoeles had made it impossible to balance in their canoes.

It is by no means just a rural disease. The unplanned growth of third world towns has produced ideal conditions—open sewers, poor drainage, inadequate housing and poor people—for the *Culex* mosquito, which thrives in urban conditions, to pass on the disease. Four decades ago two thirds of all people lived in rural communities. Today it is only just over half. By 2025, development experts expect 60% will be in urban areas. Meanwhile the *Anopheles* mosquito, which is a key LF carrier in Africa and mainly found in rural areas, can be found in small towns too. Vivian Amoah, a young attractive Ghanian, lives in Winneba, a small coastal town west of Accra. She had been training to be a financial assistant when her legs began to swell. Initially she turned to a native health healer, who cut her swollen feet with razor blades to insert herbs, only making the condition worse. She left college and now sells maize, grown by her mother, at a road junction. But she is attending a clinic, where she is learning new techniques to control the swellings.

The inspiration for the clinics is Gerusa Dreyer, a Brazilian doctor (See Chapter Six), who working on her own, cut off from the main research centres, developed new simple hygienic ways of treating the disease, which do not require highly trained medics but can be carried out by patients themselves. The LF Global Alliance has two separate and distinct prongs: the elimination of transmission campaign aimed at preventing the spread of the disease—by a mass drug treatment programme that eventually could involve treating the 1.2 billion at risk with an annual dose of two drugs for four to five years. This programme will block the transmission of the disease but not help existing patients. This is the role of the second prong: alleviating and preventing the suffering of existing patients through the simple techniques developed by Dr. Dreyer—washing and bathing the affected limbs daily with clean water, elevating the affected limbs, and simple skin care. Dr. Dreyer has also pioneered new forms of support for patients—"Hope Clubs" for the separate conditions—where the sense of self-empowerment and patient optimism is inspiring. Within patient circles, she is already regarded as a saint and a heroine. With the global campaign's help, she has produced a comprehensive guide for health workers and launched a series of international workshops training trainers so that her techniques can be quickly spread. With the help of ultrasound scans of the body, she has also pioneered new ways of diagnosing the disease that are also now being copied round the world.

The least reported patient group is perhaps the most important: children. Their infections were overlooked by earlier researchers because their clinical symptoms usually emerged in late teens or early adult years. But new research, using antigen detection tests on children's blood, show 2% are infected by the age of two and 26% by the age of four in endemic areas. The new mass drug treatment programmes that are being introduced, will not just break transmission but also kill five separate species of intestinal worms, providing an enormous boost to children's nutrition. Health researchers have shown just how seriously intestinal worms reduce physical—and intellectual—development. Under pilot trials, children's growth has been dramatically transformed. In the words of Dr. Eric Ottesen, the World Health Organization's (WHO) coordinator of the LF Global Alliance: of all LF sufferers, children stand to benefit the most from LF elimination programmes. They have their whole lives ahead of them.

Eradication campaigns have a chequered history. In the first half of the twentieth century, there was no success. The Rockefeller Foundation launched a hookworm eradication campaign in 1907 and yellow fever in 1915, but both failed. WHO tried to eliminate yaws in the late 1950s and malaria in the 1960s but failed. After each failure, scepticism towards further eradication attempts initially grew, but then subsided. The smallpox campaign, ratified by the World Health Assembly in 1966, was launched in 1967 against the opposition of sceptical critics, but within a decade, the last death from naturally contracted smallpox took place in Somalia in 1977. One of the world's deadliest diseases, that had killed millions—one out of five who contracted it suffered a harrowing death—was totally eradicated. This generated new hope for eradication. Had it not been eradicated, WHO estimates there would have been a further 350 million new victims—roughly the combined population of the U.S. and Mexico—and an estimated 40 million deaths, equivalent to the entire population of Spain and South Africa.

In the next decade, two other diseases are expected to be eradicated: polio, which has paralysed millions, was down to 3,500 new cases in 2000 in the campaign's last push; and Guinea Worm, which in the 1970s infected several million people in Africa creating the most excruciating pain as the fiery serpent burrowed its way out of the body, is now down to a few thousand thanks to a campaign coordinated by The Carter Center established by Jimmy Carter, former U.S. President in Atlanta. LF, which in some respects is an even bigger challenge than these three diseases, could be the fourth to be eradicated. The scale of the campaign is daunting. Smallpox began as a mass immunisation programme but quickly adopted a targeted approach, isolating victims and ensuring only those at risk from contact were vaccinated. Polio only involves vaccination of the under fives. LF will need to treat both children and adults—not just the 120 million infected but also the 1.2 billion at risk. Most of Nigeria's 100 million people will have to be treated. In India, the 450 million at risk will have to be reached. James Grant, the former UNICEF boss and health campaigner, declared the immunisation programmes of the 1980s were the biggest peacetime operations the world had seen. They're even bigger now. India mobilised a 2.6 million army of health workers and volunteers to achieve its National Immunisation Day target of 125 million polio vaccinations in 1999 and 2000. Mountains of ice were needed to maintain the "cold chain" to keep the vaccine cool. Transport ranged from camel trains, complete with ice packs, in remote Rajasthan to army helicopters in the Ganges valley to get round flooded roads. The LF eradication programme will not need ice—it is using drugs, not vaccines—nor will it try to reach 450 million in India in one day. But 450 million will have to be treated if the programme is to succeed. An early pilot programme involved 40 million.

The numbers are not the only challenge. The people at risk of LF are among the poorest in the world. Most are illiterate and many instinctively turn to soothsayers, witch doctors or voodoo men for what they perceive to be an affliction of an evil spirit. They find it difficult to believe the disease is spread by mosquitoes, not least because everybody in these poor communities get bitten, but not everybody gets the disease. A massive education as well as medical campaign will be needed. Success requires at least 70% to 80% of the entire at-risk community being treated. Otherwise transmission is not broken because enough infected blood will remain to keep the disease cycling via mosquitoes (See Chapter Two).

It is going to be more difficult to raise funds for LF than for the smallpox or polio campaign. Unlike smallpox or polio, LF does not threaten the developed world. Everybody in the world was at risk from smallpox until it was eliminated. It knew no limits in terms of geography, climate or vector. There was aerosol transmission—caught by inhaling the virus from an infected person. Everybody who had not been vaccinated was at risk. The dread which both diseases generated still lives on among older people in the West—the pock marks of smallpox and, even more recently, the polio threat which disabled millions and prevented many from even breathing in the first two decades after the Second World War. Until the vaccine was developed in the late 1950s, the only treatment was the "iron lung" that helped paralysed people to breathe.

LF is different. It is not fatal. Once found in temperate countries—including the U.S., Japan and China—it is now restricted to tropical zones, where the small group of mosquitoes which spread it, thrive. It requires sustained exposure—and many bites—before infection takes hold. It does not threaten the West. More complicated still, many people infected by the disease do not know they have it. Until recently, there was only one way of checking—a blood test in the middle of the night, unpopular with health workers as well as communities, many of which have no electricity.

What the elimination of LF needed was a bold and dramatic gesture. Post Second World War eradication programmes, using an early anti-filarial drug, DEC, were remarkably successful in eliminating the disease in Japan, Korea and Malaysia in the late 1950s and early 1960s. An initial programme failed in China, but it too succeeded in the 1980s. But this still left 80 states where the disease was endemic. Some developing states in Africa, the Americas and the Pacific introduced programmes, but premature relaxation of the controls led to resurgent infections. LF has become a forgotten and neglected disease, confined mainly to the poorest of the poor.

A small band of dedicated medical researchers, heavily concentrated in America but linked to field programmes in Haiti, India and the Pacific, continued to carry out control trials, but were frequently stretched for funds. Eric Ottesen, the acknowledged leading world authority, was working at the National Institute for Health in Washington, DC, the world's biggest medical research centre. Further south, at the Centers for Disease Control (CDC), the world's biggest centre specialising in disease control, there was a bigger group involving David Addiss, Pat Lammie, Thomas Streit, and Michael Beach. Japan, India and Sri Lanka had their own research teams.

None dared to think of complete eradication until two of the biggest names in public health, Bill Foege and Don Hopkins, who were involved in both the smallpox and polio campaigns, set up the International Taskforce for Disease Eradication in Atlanta with the purpose of evaluating the potential for elimination of 94 infectious diseases. Eric Ottesen was called to set out the case for the eradication of LF before the committee. In doing so he became converted. So did the taskforce. LF was identified by its high-powered members in 1993 as one of only six diseases that could be eradicated. There were three main biological and two technical reasons: humans were the only hosts, there was no multiplication of the parasite in the mosquito, the disease had a poor transmission system and good drugs and diagnostics were available. (The other five diseases identified as eradicable were: Guinea Worm, polio, mumps, rubella, and pork tape worm.) In May 1997, the World Health Assembly passed a resolution making elimination of LF a public health priority.

Out in the field, scientists were now using three different LF control drugs: DEC, a generic drug; albendazole, produced by GlaxoSmithKline (GSK); and Mectizan (ivermectin), a Merck drug which was also being used to control river blindness. Transmission of the disease occurs when microfilariae (minute, immature larvae) swimming in a patient's blood, are ingested by a mosquito, develop into larvae in the mosquito, and are passed back to another person upon the mosquito's next meal of human blood. Drugs stop the transmission by killing the millions of microfilariae in the blood, thus interrupting the transmission cycle (See Chapter Two). Albendazole is not, per se, an antifilarial drug—but enhances the transmission-breaking effect of DEC or ivermectin. In the mid 1990s, trials on dual drug programmes began.

What was still missing after the World Health Assembly vote in 1997 embracing LF eradication was any oomph. All this was changed by a celebration charity dinner in Washington in 1997, where Jan Leschly, chief executive of SmithKline Beecham before its merger with Glaxo Wellcome in 2000, sat next to former U.S. President Jimmy Carter, who had set up his own foundation campaigning to improve health. Leschly, who had turned down a British government invitation to take part in London's Dome, was looking for a bigger and more constructive millennium philanthropic project. He asked Carter if he had any ideas. Next day Carter called Bill Foege, a key adviser and the biggest name in public health. A tall, gangling friendly man, Foege's approach to public health is fired with missionary zeal. More than three decades ago, he transformed the smallpox campaign when his main supplies of the vaccine were cut off by civil war in Nigeria, where he was working. He was forced to replace mass immunisation with a targeted approach. It worked. His new strategy of surveillance and containment became widely adopted in other states. Foege has been at the heart of most of the subsequent eradication

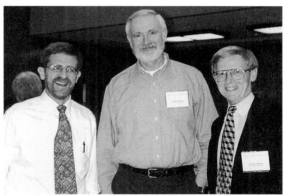

(From left to right) David Addiss, Bill Foege and Eric Ottesen at the LF Partners' Forum in Geneva, 1998.
Source: GSK

campaigns—polio, Guinea Worm, river blindness. He was a former director of the $5 billion Centers for Disease Control in the U.S. and a distinguished professor at the nearby Emory University. He has helped establish numerous task forces to reduce contagious diseases. He's also a journalist's dream, able to put complex issues simply, with an instinctive ear for a memorable metaphor or apt analogy.

It was 5:00 A.M., U.S. time. Foege was in France at a scientific meeting of the Mectizan Donation Programme, the river blindness campaign. Carter confessed to Foege he had been having difficulty sleeping. Leschly's inquiry had created too much excitement. Did he have any ideas? Serendipity had struck. Just hours before, Eric Ottesen had given the Mectizan Expert Committee the first results of the dual drug trials: instead of killing

ERIC OTTESEN:
From Academic to Global Campaign Coordinator

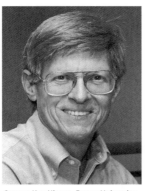

Source: Kay Hinton, Emory University

How do you change from being a dedicated scientist researching a little known disease that affects only the poorest of the poor, into a key coordinator of perhaps the biggest disease eradication campaign that has ever been launched? In his first role, Eric Ottesen lived in laboratories or in some of the remotest communities that still suffer from the disease. In his second, he has had to negotiate the complex political procedures of the big international agencies (WHO, the World Bank, UNICEF), work with the two biggest drug companies in the world, and help put together a public/private alliance of more than 30 different parties each with their own culture.

Challenged to explain how he has coped, Eric Ottesen produces one of his familiar rueful grins and an equally familiar honest answer: "With difficulty. It has been like living in a whirlwind. Everything moves. But what an immensely rewarding experience with so much progressing on so many fronts."

Dr. Ottesen set out to be an academic. A brilliant teacher at his first university, Princeton, ignited his interest in biology, but he went on to Harvard medical school and a further two years at the pediatrics department of Duke. On graduation from this 10 years of study, rather than accept the Vietnam draft, he opted instead to enter public health at the National Institutes for Health (NIH) in Washington. He was to stay there for 22 years.

He moved into the study of filarial worms (there are nine, of which six cause diseases) and found almost no one studying lymphatic filariasis (LF). He explains: "It wasn't applicable to western people. There was no one left with the disease. There were other challenges. It was difficult to set up experimental models—it didn't work in mice. There was an enormously long cycle. Access to patients was difficult. But with almost no one studying it, it meant there was no competition. It was an open field."

Thirty years later there are many more scientists in the field but Ottesen is the acknowledged world authority. He carries his immense knowledge lightly. He is open, friendly and has an infectious laugh. He is also a brilliant teacher as this reporter can testify. I arrived in Geneva knowing little about the disease, but was patiently given my first tour through the medical labyrinth.

Ottesen moved from NIH to WHO to take charge of filarial control in 1994 never suspecting the whirlwind which was going to hit him. He had planned to continue his scientific work alongside his WHO work.

Fortunately Ottesen has that other key characteristic for public health workers: optimism. Whenever I have come back from my various trips and expressed doubts about the daunting scale of the enterprise, nothing but positive responses get uttered down his end of the telephone: "Look, everyone is benefiting. The children are healthier with fewer worms and lice. The adults feel better. The community is stronger from taking part in the programme and helping to rid itself of the disease. National politicians have seen the advantages of promoting it. The programme has a momentum of its own."

He is even more positive about the LF Global Alliance. He is particularly excited by the way the different partners are working together in spite of their different cultures: "This is a partnership that is going to get even better and it is good now. Of course there are going to be setbacks. But it is more than strong enough to weather them."

Dr. Ottesen is moving back to the U.S. from Geneva in the second half of 2001. There he will help co-ordinate the LF work of the three key Atlanta agencies—Emory, CDC and the Carter Center. It will also allow him to work as a bridge between WHO and the U.S. There has always been tension between WHO and the U.S., not least because of the giant American institutions for disease control with budgets five times as large as WHO's. LF needs all parties to pull together.

80% to 90% of microfilariae, dual drug doses were achieving 99%. There could not have been a more obvious project for GlaxoSmithKline—their drug was a key player. It not only enhanced the performance of the other two drugs, but albendazole is an even more effective killer of the five main species of intestinal worms. David Addiss, a scientist at the Centers for Disease Control, was at the French meeting. He described what happened when Foege returned to the room after Carter's telephone call: "There was a twinkle in his eye and anticipation and excitement in the room as we waited to see if we would be told what was said. We threw several ideas around, but albendazole was a clear winner. Foege was all too aware of how the Merck donation of Mectizan for river blindness had transformed that campaign. He had always hoped that this highly successful public/private partnership on disease control could act as a model for future replication. Now here was the chance."

Even before the Leschly and Carter talks, GSK scientists had become aware of the dual drug trials which had opened up a new role for albendazole: eradicating LF. Two GSK scientists, Dr. John Horton and Manouchehr Yazhari, were at an American Society of Tropical Medicine conference in California where Eric Ottesen had presented the same findings that he later delivered to the Mectizan Donation meeting in France. Eric Ottesen, describes the reactions of the GSK scientists: They were genuinely excited about this new role. Until then, albendazole had only been marketed as an extremely effective de-worming pill. Horton, who had a long association with the drug and Yazhari, who was responsible for community health programme sales in the developing world, went back to London to talk to company vice presidents, including the genial Dr. James Hill, head of corporate relations. Albendazole donations became one option for the company's millennium project. Yazhari went to WHO headquarters and made crucial early contacts with the director of its CTD (Control of Tropical Diseases) division, Dr. Kazem Behbehani, who became a convert to the cause and promptly found more money to save the dual drug trials that were facing financial collapse.

Carter invited Leschly and senior GSK executives to meet Foege and other health officials at the Atlanta-based Carter Center. At that time, only one pharmaceutical company was making serious donations of drugs for third world diseases: Merck, which had donated 100 million doses of Mectizan over a decade in the fight against river blindness in Africa. Leschly, along with Dr. James Hill and a small group of other GSK scientists, flew down to Atlanta. Foege describes the Atlanta meeting thus: "It was an unforgettable event. Here were these senior business people with real corporate power asking how they could put their influence to social good. It was quite different to the picture we held about chief executives at that time. They were clearly serious about trying to use their influence, beyond making profits for their shareholders, to create social capital."

The initial talk at the meeting centred on what GSK could do to eradicate measles. Foege explained the difficulties faced by such a campaign. At that point, Dr. Hill put up the idea of an albendazole donation—a proposal both sides had reached by separate routes. GSK agreed to provide free albendazole tablets over 20 years for a dual drug programme that could require the 1.2 billion people at risk to take annual doses for four to five years. Ottesen, who was in charge of LF control at WHO, points to three key midwives involved in the birth of the eradication campaign: James Hill, Manouchehr Yazhari and Kazem Behbehani. Once born, it was Ottesen and Brian Bagnall, who became GSK's LF director, who had to nursemaid it through its infancy.

Thus emerged what London's Financial Times has described as "the biggest single act of corporate philanthropy in any industry". GSK went to talk to the top officials of the World Health Organization (WHO). There, at their eight-storey headquarters in a 17-acre park on the outskirts of Geneva, negotiations went smoothly. A U.N. agency with 191 member states, WHO has played the leading role in the eradication and control of infectious diseases since 1948. In December, 1997, just four months before WHO's 50th birthday, GSK and WHO signed a Memorandum of Understanding on a joint campaign to eliminate LF. The

WHO/GSK announcement was welcomed by the World Bank's president, James Wolfensohn, who with other U.N. family members were invited by WHO's director general to join in. The LF Global Alliance, which now numbers 37 partners, was beginning to roll. Albendazole, one of the two drugs needed in the annual dual dose, would be donated free by the company. DEC, which costs less than $0.005 per dose (92 cents per 200 patients), will be used as the second drug. It cannot be used in Africa, where it would be a threat to patients because of its effects on other parasites they carry, but Merck came to the rescue here. Already heavily committed to free donations of Mectizan for the river blindness campaign, the company agreed to donate Mectizan to the even greater numbers of LF sufferers. In a unique dual drug company philanthropic deal, it has agreed to donate all the ivermectin that will be needed on the African continent. This was a remarkable development in corporate philanthropy. Here was Merck, the world's second biggest drug company, already running at that time the biggest philanthropic programme, ready to join a second and even more demanding philanthropic programme, launched by its biggest competitor.

Oomph had finally arrived with the GSK and Merck donations. The lonely researchers, who had doggedly continued with their research into what was the most unfashionable of diseases, suddenly but deservedly found themselves on sunny uplands. For years they limped along on the smallest of grants, in some of the most inhospitable climates, with seemingly little chance of international recognition. Asked why they were so nice—and so patient in explaining the intricacies of the disease to this reporter—David Addiss of the CDC summed it up well: "There is no room for prima donnas in this field. We are working with the poorest of the poor. There was no room for international recognition when we started. If you wanted a Nobel prize you'd be better advised to concentrate on the acute conditions challenging the West." Yet now, these same committed and intelligent researchers, thanks to the LF Global Alliance, find themselves at the forefront of a pioneering eradication programme.

The creation of the alliance was crucial. Foege is unequivocal about the future of eradication programmes: they will only succeed if they can create large coalitions of international organisations, private pharmaceutical companies, voluntary organisations and research institutes. He points to the huge support effort that is needed—transport, training, distribution, epidemiological surveillance, community education—that is needed on top of free drugs. Part of the polio success story was getting the support of Rotary, the international service club, which not only raised $400 million for the campaign, but even more important, had members in key positions round the world able to lobby government and officials in support of the campaign. It was Rotary members in India who helped persuade the Indian government to go for the mass immunisation days by organising a successful pilot in Delhi. The river blindness campaign is a coalition of Merck, the Mectizan Donation Program, plus the WHO, the World Bank, numerous international agencies, Ministries of Health, more than 30 non-governmental development organisations, international donors, and local health workers.

Dr. Gro Harlem Brundtland, the feisty former Prime Minister of Norway and leading environmentalist who took over as WHO Director General in July, 1998, is equally unequivocal about such coalitions: "Some people have suggested that industry-WHO partnerships such as the LF Global Alliance, represent a conflict of interest. On the contrary, we believe such collaboration which provides drugs for periods long enough to reach the target, are an exemplary commitment to public health in the 21st century." Brian Bagnall, the GSK director with responsibility for LF, was the key GSK player working with WHO officials to put the alliance together. He is passionate about the campaign, is an astute judge of character and, crucially, is able to recognise the pressures and restraints which other organisations are undergoing. (See profile in Chapter Seven).

The LF Global Alliance is an impressive coalition of 37 bodies including three international organisations (WHO, World Bank, UNICEF); the two pharmaceutical multinationals (GSK and Merck); seven national aid agencies (Australia, Belgium, Italy, Japan, the Netherlands, Spain, U.S. plus the Arab Fund for Economic and Social Development); eight non-governmental organisations including the Carter Center in the U.S. and Health and Development International, Norway; two powerful and prestigious academic institutions, the Liverpool School of Tropical Medicine and Emory University's Rollins School of Public Health in Atlanta; the world's biggest organisation for fighting infectious diseases, CDC (Centers for Disease Control) in Atlanta; plus the Ministries of Health of Endemic Countries (see full list of partners at end of Chapter Seven).

The first meeting of the Alliance partners at Santiago de Compostela in Spain in May, 2000, demonstrated the momentum and goodwill that had been created. GSK has been helping with training, research, surveys and planning. Both GSK and Merck are helping with transport. Yet more funds are still needed. Dr. Anne Haddix, an economist at the Rollins School of Public Health told a London conference convened by the Royal Society of Tropical Medicine and Hygiene in January 2000, that on top of $400 million in free drug donations provided by GSK and Merck for the first five years of the programme, a further $600 million would be needed to cover support costs.

A big boost to the LF Global Alliance came with the announcement in late 2000 of a $20 million donation over five years from the Bill and Melinda Gates Foundation towards the eradication campaign. After the drug donations from GSK and Merck, this is the single biggest donation the Alliance has received. The money is being divided between four parties: WHO; the Atlanta complex that includes Emory, the Carter Center and CDC; the NDGOs working in the field; and the Liverpool School of Tropical Medicine for its support work across the campaign. Ingeniously, the Gates Foundation left it to the four parties to decide how the total should be divided up. A three-day conference in Chester, England, in January 2001, chaired by Dr. Bernhard Liese of the World Bank, which is acting as banker for the donation, reached a consensus on how it should be spent. A key area on which Gates money will focus is on finding the best way of reaching the 70% to 80% of the at-risk community that has to be treated if transmission is to be broken.

A Gates Grant Review Committee, with representatives from all four groups, has been set up. In addition to the priorities of the four parties, cross party priorities include alleviation and prevention of LF by simple local treatment methods pioneered by Dr. Dreyer; research to demonstrate to nation states the economic benefits of the eradication programme; surveys of successful LF elimination pilot projects, justifying a scaling up of the programme to a national level. Observers at the Chester meeting, expressed delight at how the Gates money, which might have led to division between the parties, brought the LF Global Alliance closer together. The message was clear: the Alliance is working.

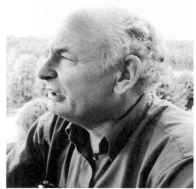

David Molyneux, LF Support Centre at Liverpool School of Tropical Medicine. Source: GSK

Both Brian Bagnall and Eric Ottesen pay tribute to the two academic institutions—in Liverpool and Emory —that have been working within the Alliance. They speak of them helping to provide bridges between the many different member organisations and supplying the glue that has allowed the Alliance to gel. The Liverpool School, under the direction of Dr. David Molyneux, has worked across a broad

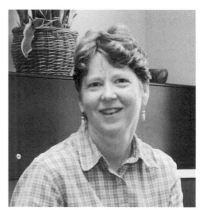

Anne Haddix, LF Support Center, Emory University. Source: Kay Hinton, Emory University

front including back up support for mapping exercises (monitoring the extent of the disease), training workshops and preparing strategy papers. They are helping to ensure the annual £1m donation from the UK's Department for International Development (DFID) reaches the hands of people who both need it and can use it. Brian Bagnall pays tribute to Molyneux's "knowledge, fairness and strategic vision."

The Emory effort, guided by Dr. Anne Haddix, has produced a series of papers on the projected cost of the campaign and the economic benefits that eradication of LF will generate. They are providing invaluable ammunition for health ministries to use in persuading national governments to endorse the international campaign. An early paper for the World Bank demonstrated the benefits of integrating LF elimination with the river blindness campaign in West Africa. The piggy back option, guided by the Carter Center in Nigeria, under which two or even three (LF, river blindness and schistosomiasis) campaigns share costs, offer dramatic savings (See Chapter Five). Just integrating LF with APOC's river blindness campaign in Africa would save $62 million over 20 years and have a 28% economic rate of return. Other Emory studies are looking at the cost effectiveness of integrating LF with community-directed health programmes, malaria bednet initiatives and the economic benefits which Dr. Dreyer's treatment clinics generate for local and national economies.

Like all eradication campaigns, LF has had its hiccups in its first three years. The GSK/WHO deal coincided with a much-needed reorganisation of WHO, pushed through by the determined Dr. Brundtland. Her predecessor, Dr. Hiroshi Nakajima, was widely criticised for mismanagement and poor focus. This inevitably led to delays as the CTD (Control of Tropical Diseases) division was reorganised and placed in the newly created Communicable Disease Cluster, under the experienced hands of Dr. David Heymann. An epidemiologist whose experiences stretch back to India's smallpox campaign in the 1970s, Dr. Heymann has extensive experience of sub-Saharan Africa and has published over 100 scientific articles on infectious diseases. Few are better qualified, but the initial delays caused frustration in the ranks of public health workers, eager to begin their LF campaign.

Safety tests caused a second hiccup. Tens of millions of people have used ivermectin; hundreds of millions DEC and albendazole. But only tens of thousands had been involved in the dual drug trials. Did a dual dose, when so many had separately used both and the dual trials far exceeded the numbers used in a normal testing of a drug, require an exhaustive review? The scientists were divided but a exhaustive review was given the go ahead. A systematic review of all research studies was undertaken by two separate teams. What emerged was a safety procedure which will convince the most sceptical of critics. As Eric Ottesen noted in Spain, the Alliance has emerged from these challenges in strengthened form.

Cheering on from the sidelines is Bill Foege. He likes the way the LF campaign has begun without years of pre-planning: "There is no point in waiting to define all the barriers before starting because most of the barriers will only be found after the start of the programme. If you wait until you know everything, you simply don't do anything."

Foege urges the campaign to concentrate on recruiting optimists. Pessimists and cynics were not just wrong about smallpox but harmful. They diverted attention, generated doubts in potential donors, invented problems far beyond the vast array of existing ones. "Even though negative views can be of value, their usefulness is limited. Large problems require optimism." He quotes Schweitzer on Africa, "This continent needs people who never become doubters", and points to the 1993 World Bank study that reported health had improved more in the last 40 years than in all of recorded history. This was still true, despite the advent of AIDS and resurgence in some other infective diseases. He notes: "Two decades ago, measles was the single most dangerous virus killing three million a year. Today it kills one million, which is far too many, but look at the progress."

Foege notes that the smallpox alliance, jointly promoted by the U.S./U.S.S.R. in 1966 was at the height of the Cold War: "If we could form this alliance during the cold war, how many alliances can we form now?" He points to the growing involvement of the pharmaceutical industry in public eradication programmes. On top of river blindness and LF, there are three other drug donation programmes: Pfizer in a new campaign against trachoma, the debilitating eye disease; Novartis, the Swiss company, with drugs for leprosy; and GSK with a second drug donation programme involving an anti malarial drug.

Foege adds: "Future generations will look back to the last four decades in as much awe at the breakthroughs in disease control, as we look back today to the architects and builders who created the cathedrals of 900 years ago—remember, Europe was rewarded with not just cathedrals but much better building techniques for all structures. What society is doing now is creating equivalent public health cathedrals, which through diagnostic, treatment and surveillance programmes, will improve public health across the board."

CHAPTER TWO

How the Cause of LF Was Discovered—And With It, Tropical Medicine

Patrick Manson, the doctor who is internationally recognised as "the father" of tropical medicine, first made his name working as a physician in a remote Chinese port, where he identified the blood-sucking mosquito as the key agent in the transmission of lymphatic filariasis (LF) in 1877. He went on to make a host of other discoveries, but his first discovery remained his most important by opening a new door in medicine. A succession of other diseases were later shown to be transmitted by blood-sucking insects, among them malaria (1898), yellow fever (1900) dengue (1903) and onchocerciasis, otherwise known as river blindness.

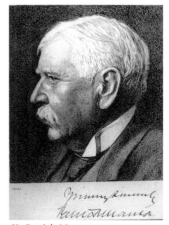

Sir Patrick Manson
Source: Wellcome Trust Library

Manson's achievement would have been historic even in a modern setting, but was phenomenal given the primitive conditions under which he was working. Less than a year after graduating as a doctor in Aberdeen in 1865, he joined the Chinese Imperial Maritime Customs, serving first in Formosa (now Taiwan) for five years and then another 12 years in Amoy, a "treaty port" on the mainland, established soon after the Opium War. Officially the service was a branch of the Peking government, but it was led and heavily staffed by the British. As a medical officer, he was expected "to inspect ships calling at the port and treat their crews". But having unbounded energy, he developed a private practice (for the Chinese as well as the few Europeans), helped out in missionary hospitals for poor Chinese patients, and conducted extensive private research into the multiple number of diseases that surrounded his practice: leprosy, malaria, smallpox, dengue, cholera, typhoid, beriberi, paragonomiasis.

But it was LF which particularly attracted him in his early days. Through his own and the missionary hospitals' patients, he quickly became familiar with both elephantiasis and hydrocoele, for which he conducted surgical corrections. He was appalled by the gross physical deformities generated by the disease. Amoy, which was described by contemporaries as "redolent with every impurity" and "superlatively filthy", was a difficult place in which to conduct research. There was little intellectual stimulation, no scientists off whom he could bounce ideas, few books, no museum, no scientific meetings or critical colleagues. Manson wrote to Spencer Cobbold, the leading British parasitologist of the day: "I live in an out-of-the-world place away from libraries, out of the run of what is going on, so I do not know the value of my work, or if it has been done before, or better." He even confessed: "Men like myself in general practice are but poor and slow investigators crippled as we are by the necessity of making our daily bread."

Even so, research is what the indefatigable physician did conduct at length. In 1875 he returned to Britain on leave. Having no access to London's scientific circles, he went to the British Museum instead, where Karl Marx was another busy burrower in its library, writing his Das Kapital, the book that prompted the Russian revolution and promoted international communism. In another part of the library, Manson discovered the writings of Timothy Lewis, another Aberdeen graduate, serving in India with the Army Medical Service, where he had discovered microfilaria (MF) in the urine of chyluria patients. Chyluria is a condition in which lymphatic fluid leaks into urine turning it white. Lewis also examined the blood of the patients finding MF there too. He concluded that MF were an embryonic larvae of a much larger adult nematode worm. He suggested all patients suffering from obscure diseases should have their blood examined.

Manson seized on this proposal returning to China with a new and much more powerful microscope as well as a new wife. On his arrival he conducted a succession of studies on blood from diseased and healthy patients, on urine from patients suffering from chyluria, on the lymph tissue from hydrocoele patients, and on tissue from elephantiasis. He showed that 10% of the population suffered from LF and this increased with age up to 30% for people over 70. He believed the different conditions of LF—chyluria, hydrocoele, elephantiasis—had a single pathological state and in October 1880, he found and described a parent worm alive and active in the lymphatic system.

Unknown to Manson he was not the first to discover an adult worm. Joseph Bancroft, a British doctor who had migrated to Brisbane, Australia, had found one in an abscess in 1876. And Lewis turned out not to be the first to discover microfilaria in urine. This was discovered by Otto Wucherer, a German physician working in Brazil, six years earlier than Lewis. Thus the parasite was given the generic name of *Wuchereria* and the adult parasite *Wuchereria bancrofti.* But Manson was the first to establish that the adult worm was a parasite of the lymphatic system.

Having established that there were adult worms, male and female, in the lymphatic system producing microfilariae, Manson was fascinated about their purpose. He concluded the millions in a person's blood could not possibly mature in the host without killing the person—"an anomaly impossible in nature." He concluded there must be an intermediary and after rejecting fleas, bugs, lice and sandflies, intuitively opted for the blood-sucking mosquito.

In a clinical experiment, Manson, whose ethics would cause apoplexy among modern medical ethicists, used his Chinese servant, Hin Loo, whose blood already had an established high concentration of microfilariae, to act as a human guinea pig. He placed him on a bench at night in a square wooden frame (10 by 6.5 ft), that was covered with fine mosquito-gauze, left the door open for 30 minutes with a light to attract mosquitoes, and the next morning caught the engorged insects and dissected them. He found a high concentration of MF in their stomachs. (Over a century later, researchers mapping the prevalence of the disease, do something similar: they fumigate the huts in which native people are living and dissect the mosquitoes that drop dead, to determine how many are carrying MF.)

Manson described his experiment: "I shall not easily forget the first mosquito I dissected. I tore off its abdomen and succeeded in expressing the blood the stomach contained. . . ." Even more interestingly, he discovered the parasite had metamorphosed from "a simple structureless animal" into a much bigger and formidable creature having "developed a mouth, an alimentary canal and other organs . . . manifestly it was on the road to a new human host."

He had established that the transmission required a cycle of development in the mosquito and even at that time, 1887, recognised the potential for eradication by noting "from the fact of the disease depending on so tangible a link . . . it is quite possible to prevent its spread, if not to secure its extermination". His observations were sent to Spencer Cobbold, who ensured they were written up by the *Lancet*, the British medical journal in 1878, as well as communicated to a London medical society, the Linnean Society, of which he was president.

But Manson had not got everything right. He was working at a time when it was assumed mosquitoes only bit once, obtained blood, and died five days later. This led Manson to assume that transmission occurred through humans drinking infected water, with the third stage larvae escaping as the dying mosquito landed on water to lay her eggs. What he hadn't realised was that the advanced larvae he found in his dissection was not from the meal provided by Hin Loo, but from earlier blood meals the mosquitoes had consumed.

It was not until 1900 that C.G. Low, a scientist working under Manson and alongside Joseph Bancroft's son Thomas, was able to show that infected larvae within the mosquito eventually migrate to its proboscis. Using a new technique that was able to cut the mosquito's proboscis in half, they found two infected larvae there waiting for the mosquito to take a second bite. Manson believed the larvae developed within seven days inside the mosquito. We now know that MF in blood ingested by a mosquito takes between 10 and 20 days to develop into an "infective larvae" (called L3 by the scientists). The entire transmission system is very "inefficient", which is another reason why LF's potential for eradication is high.

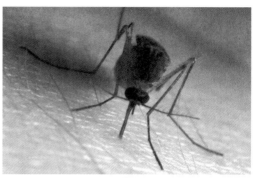

Mosquito completes the life cycle of LF by ingesting microfilariae in blood that are later transformed into infective larvae and deposited on skin during feeding
Source: WHO/TDR

The female mosquito (the male does not bite) sucks human blood for protein for her eggs. The chances of MF being in blood that a mosquito sucks depends on the level of infection in the area and the individual. But even when a mosquito ingests MF—it

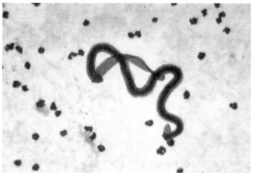

Microfilaria in blood
Source: WHO/TDR/Wellcome

only requires 1–2 micro litres of blood—there is still only a 50:50 chance that the MF will survive to become an infective parasite. Mosquitoes only live between 7 and 21 days, depending on the weather and predators. The LF parasite takes between 10 and 20 days to develop, thus many die within the mosquito before the parasite matures into an infective larvae. Mature larvae that survive, migrate from the mosquito's stomach into the flight muscles in the shoulders and finally to the insect's mouth parts. When the mosquito takes its next blood meal, the active larvae crawl on to the surface of the victim's skin and tries to enter the body through the tiny feeding hole left by the mosquito. If there is low humidity, the larvae dies on the skin, unable to reach the feeding holes.

Once back inside a human host, the larvae migrate to the lymphatic system, the network of nodes and vessels that provide the body with crucial defences against infection and cancer. The lymphatic system collects the watery fluid (lymph) that all body tissues are bathed in, and helps transport it back to the heart to flow back into the bloodstream. Lymph plays a key role in the immune system. The nodes in the lymphatic system act as filters, trapping microorganisms and other foreign bodies in the lymph. The nodes contain a type of white blood cell which can neutralize or destroy invading bacteria and viruses. If part of the body becomes diseased or inflamed, the nearby lymph nodes become swollen and tender as they limit the spread of the disease. Compared to blood vessels, the circulatory lymphatic system is much more delicate. The vessels are extremely thin. The system does not have a pump, like the heart, to move its fluid. Instead it is moved by muscles and held by valves.

It takes the larvae between 3 and 12 months to grow into thread-like parasitic filarial worms. Both male and female worms are needed to produce microfilariae. They mate in nests, which Gerusa Dreyer (See Chapter Six) successfully identified with the use of ultrasound. Each female produces millions of MF. They can live for up to seven years or more. Females grow to 10cm, males to only 4cm. A typical patient will have two or three nests but 15 nests have been found by Dr. Dreyer. They congregate inside the scrotal sac in males, where it is cooler. The average nest will have two to three worms but the largest had 26 females and two males. There are normally five females for every male.

The precise damage which the parasite causes to the lymphatic system is still unclear. Scientists like Eric Ottesen believe the worms may secrete a substance, which causes the valves in the lymphatic system to dilate. Other scientists, like Dr. Dreyer, believe the microfilariae cause damage too. Whatever the cause, the smooth passage of immune fluid round the system gets interrupted. It no longer clears itself. The circulation of immune cells, which are needed to clear up infections, is interrupted. Pools collect and lymphoedema develops (swelling in the legs, arms, breasts and genitals). Further trouble can be caused when the worm dies, and the system is unable to clear the obstruction, or drain itself properly. This challenge faces the eradication campaign. One of the drugs, DEC, can kill about half the worms in a human host; this causes short term problems for patients as their lymphatic systems deal with the obstructions.

Manson's discoveries did not stop at identifying the mosquito as a key transmission agent. A second discovery was the "nocturnal periodicity" of MF—the fact that they disappear from human blood during daylight hours, but reappear and reach peak density in the middle of the night, coinciding with mosquito feeding habits. Manson wrote to Cobbold: "It is marvellous how Nature has adapted the habits of Filaria to those of the mosquito. . . ." Cobbold was equally delighted at "embryos, with almost military punctuality, marching to their nocturnal quarters. . . ." Others, initially, met this discovery with complete disbelief. Later researchers were to discover that in parts of the Pacific, where there are daylight biting mosquitoes, MF circulate during daylight hours but not at night.

A third Manson discovery was the great variation among mosquito species of the likelihood of spreading LF. Of four separate species in Amoy, only one, *Culex quinquefasciatus* was spreading the disease. We now know of the 3,500 species of mosquito in the world, *Culex quinquefasciatus* plus half-a-dozen species drawn from three other groups, *Anopheles, Aedes* and *Mansonia*, account for 99% of LF.

To make things marginally more complicated, *Wuchereria bancrofti* is not the only form of LF, although it accounts for 90% of the disease. *Brugia malayi* (brugian filariasis) is spread by

Mansonia mosquitoes in South Asia and accounts for most of the other 10%. *Brugia timori,* spread by an *Anopheles* mosquito, restricted to just two Indonesian islands, Flores and Timor, makes up the rest.

Manson's discoveries were not confined to LF. He played a key role in the world of Ronald Ross, who subsequently won the second Nobel prize in medicine, for his research in India showing how malaria was being transmitted by mosquitoes. Manson had long suspected the mosquito as the agent in the transmission of malaria. Ross sought out Manson in 1894, when both were back in London, and was encouraged by Manson to continue his study of the disease as a member of the Indian medical service. Like Manson in his earlier days in China, Ross felt isolated in India. He wrote Manson 110 letters of roughly 1,000 words each between April, 1895 and February, 1899, and received long replies to each.

Manson moved from Amoy to Hong Kong in 1883, where as well as continuing his work as a physician and researcher, he set up the medical school which is now part of Hong Kong university. He returned to Scotland, aged 45, with the intention of retiring on his substantial savings, but fortunately for tropical medicine, the value of the Chinese dollar collapsed. He was forced to return to work, moving to London where he practised as a physician, held a position at the Albert Dock Hospital, and began to lecture on tropical medicine at Charing Cross and St. George's hospitals.

Soon after being appointed medical adviser to the colonial office, he began to lobby for the reform of medical education in Britain, which at the time—despite the large number of civil servants and administrators being sent out to the colonies—did not include tropical medicine. He found an eager ally in Joseph Chamberlain, who as Colonial Secretary was shocked to discover the death rate of his overseas staff. In Ghana alone, 28% of 176 serving European officers ended their careers in 1896 from death or ill health.

Manson's lobbying eventually led to the creation of Britain's two tropical medicine schools—Liverpool, which opened in

May, 1899, and London, that admitted its first students in October, 1900. By then Manson had published his Manual of Tropical Diseases, which established tropical medicine as a distinct medical specialty in 1898. He subsequently had huge numbers of national and international honours bestowed on him and became the first President of the Royal Society of Tropical Medicine in 1907. Appropriately, it was the Royal Society which hosted the international conference in January, 2000, where the first countries to initiate LF eradication programmes were announced—and it is the Liverpool School, under its former director David Molyneux, which is providing key support services for the frontline campaign teams. (See Chapter Seven).

Eli Chernin, the Harvard academic, sums up Manson well: "His ingenuity would have been remarkable had he been working in the stimulating atmosphere of London or Paris, but alone in Amoy in the late 1870s, Manson's originality boggles the mind. Carlyle would surely have included him among his 'inventive men'."

This chapter is indebted to the following studies:

1. The essay by G. C. Cook, consultant physician, Hospital for Tropical Diseases, London, on the emergence of Dr. Patrick Manson on the London medical scene in "From the Greenwich hulks to Old St Pancras", the Athlone Press, 1992.
2. The third Manson oration delivered by Ian McGregor of the Liverpool School of Tropical Medicine, published by the *Royal Society of Tropical Medicine and Hygiene* (1995).
3. Eli Chernin's "Patrick Manson (1844–1922) and the transmission of filariasis", the *American Journal of Tropical Medicine and Hygiene,* 1977.
4. Eli Chernin's historical article, "Sir Patrick Manson's Studies on Transmission and Biology of Filariasis," *Reviews of Infectious Diseases,* vol 5 no 1, January–February, 1983, the University of Chicago.
5. *Patrick Manson,* the biography written by his medical son-in-law, Sir Philip Manson-Bahr, published by Thomas Nelson, 1962.

CHAPTER THREE

Village Life— And Community Health Campaigns

AFRICA

The scene could not have looked more idyllic. The sandy tree-shaded track led us down to a pale blue lagoon. Beyond the lagoon, a ridge of silver sand heavily dotted with coconut palms, stretched in either direction. Beneath the palms, peeping up from the far side of the silver ridge, was a long romantic line of thatched roofs. Beyond them was a deep blue sea. It could have been an exotic tourist development in Florida, Kenya or the Seychelles. The picturesque position would certainly have conformed with every developer's dream. But these were not imitation African huts, complete with hot and cold running water, air conditioning and luxurious bathrooms. These were genuine African huts with dirt floors, mud walls, holes for windows, no running water, no flushing loos, no electricity, no carpets, no curtains, not even any mosquito nets to protect the inhabitants from the nightly invasion of the blood-sucking vectors from the surrounding savannah.

An elderly naked man, washing himself in the lagoon, was clearly embarrassed by the arrival of two four-wheel drive vehicles spilling out health workers. The meaning of the village's name, Worabeba ("You have to desire to come"), quickly became apparent. Two children, no more than eight years old, in the bright brown and yellow uniforms worn by Ghanaian pupils, walked past us and without stopping began wading across the lagoon to their homes. The water was quickly up to their chests. A mother with a baby on her back and a large metal bowl filled with vegetables on her head, followed and soon overtook the children.

The Gulf of Guinea provides the villagers of Worabeba with plenty of fish but for everything else, they have to wade across to Ensuakyir, the village on the inland side of the lagoon. Ensuakyir does not look as romantic. It has breeze block homes, as well as traditional huts with walls made from bamboo poles and mud, thatched with a roof of palm fronds. Cooking is carried out in separate nearby thatched huts, with a small fire in one corner and clay oven by its side. It relieves the living huts of the smoke. Some families had kerosene stoves, but the kerosene had to be bought and brought from town.

The sign about Ensuakyir community centre reads "Eye Papa, A eye ma woho" (if you do good, you do it for yourself). The village chief knew we were coming. The hard bare soil near his house had been swept. A large settee and chairs had been brought out and arranged in a square. We met under the shade of acacia trees with the chief and his elders along one side, we visitors along another, village people and children filling the other places. Inquisitive small goats, chickens and bantams looked on.

The chief told us about the other side of the idyllic picture— the lack of transport, the low earnings which put even bicycles out of reach of most families, the limited farming potential of Ghana's coastal savannah. They were able to grow groundnuts (peanuts), cassava, okra and beans. They enjoyed the fruits of date and coconut palms, but were unable to grow them commercially. There was no village health centre. The nearest transport was three miles down the dirt track.

Disease was the biggest enemy. Samuel Odoom, the district disease officer in charge of 180 villages, gave us some figures. Villagers had suffered from a succession of diseases: malaria, onchocerciasis (river blindness), Guinea Worm, yaws, schistosomiasis (bilharzia), measles, whooping cough and lymphatic filariasis (LF). Some battles were being won. No paralytic polio had been recorded since 1971. Guinea worm was down to five cases compared to 600 in the past. River blindness had been dramatically cut. They were ready to embark on a LF elimination campaign.

In a typical sub Saharan African village, 260 out of every 1,000 villagers are infected with LF. About 75 of the 500 men in the village will be affected by hydrocoele. On average the village will lose between 3% and 10% of its productive labour. An impoverished community is made even more impoverished.

The villagers of Ensuakyir were in urgent need of bed nets, impregnated with insecticide, to protect themselves from disease-carrying mosquitoes. But each net cost £5, which was more than two-thirds of the villagers' weekly income. There were few nets in the village. One reason for the high price was a 25% import duty. Later, when I met the acting health minister, Dr. Moses Adiho, who had earlier served as director of health, he justified the duty on the grounds that current nets were all imported. The government was trying to get them produced locally. Ironically, other health officials told me the cloth would still have to be imported and Ghana's labour costs were likely to make the cost of home-produced nets even higher. Meanwhile Ensuakyir, one of 650 villages in Ghana which suffers from both LF and malaria, is missing one of the most effective ways of reducing both diseases.

THE PACIFIC

Just how effective bed nets can be has been demonstrated on the other side of the world by health workers in Vanuatu, the former New Hebrides that was run jointly by the British and French. A Y-shaped archipelago of 83 tropical islands, 64 of which are inhabited, Vanuatu stretches across 1,000 km of Pacific ocean just south of the Solomon islands. The total population is only 200,000. Research studies in Africa have suggested people in heavily endemic areas can suffer 100 mosquito bites in a night. One Pacific study more than doubled that number.

Vanuatu has even more people living in rural communities than Ghana—75% of its population, as against 65% in the African state. There are about 3,000 villages, a large proportion with fewer than 50 people in them, distributed mostly along narrow coastal strips or on offshore islets. The last census showed 50% of the people are living in communities of between 10 and 50 people and 25% in even smaller groups. Like Ghana, rural life in Vanuatu provides health workers with an invaluable social structure still in place. Melanesian by descent, many of the people have little sense of nationhood. Like many remote communities, the rural people identify with their village, rather than their island, let alone the 83 islands that make up the state of Vanuatu.

Any health campaign has to be decentralised by the nature of such a society. That is how the LF campaign (See Chapter Four) is being run in Vanuatu. Senior health officials provide a framework but leave many key decisions, such as how the drugs should be distributed, to local community workers. And that was how Vanuatu's anti-malaria campaign, which distributed bed nets that have also helped reduce LF, worked. The nets were distributed free of charge to vulnerable people (pregnant women, children under five, people over 60 and the disabled) with a small charge levied on the rest of the community. Regularly impregnated with insecticide, which lasts between six and 12 months, the nets kill most mosquitoes that land and prevent those that survive from biting the humans underneath. The nets have helped cut the incidence of malaria by more than four-fifths, from 17,000 cases in 1989 to 3,000 in 1998. The scheme is being run alongside a much more active mosquito control programme. As the mosquito that spreads malaria on the islands is the same that spreads LF, the LF campaign had achieved lift-off even before its formal launch in the summer of 2000. St. Valentine's Day on Vanuatu is anti-mosquito day. Even the Prime Minister gets involved, brushing out his backyard to ensure there are no places for mosquitoes to lurk.

Vanuatu's island communities may be poor but a well-tiered health structure is in place. At the lowest level are aid posts. Saama, a fishing and farming village on the main island of Efate, has only

32 households but contains an aid post in a red and white hut, made out of platted bamboo with a palm frond roof. It includes one bed as well as a cupboard with basic medicines. There is a volunteer health worker and a brightly decorated hut next door, providing sleeping accommodation for the family or friends of sick outlying farming families, who come in for treatment.

Mele, several miles farther along the coast road, provided a good example of a middle tier dispensary. Under the endearing signpost Fare Maurifaga (the house that gives health), nurse Lehi Lucy has been running it for 28 years. She has two assistants for a village of 272 households. She showed me her extensive records on every family in the village and the surrounding countryside. A decade ago 40 patients a year came to her with malaria. Last year there were only four. Life is looking up for the villagers, whose small gardens crammed with fruit trees—grapefruit, guava, paw paw, lime, breadfruit, and a variety of nut trees—suggest they do not suffer from a vitamin deficiency.

Paonangisu health centre is at the top of the primary care tree—with treatment rooms, separate maternity unit and accommodation for two nurses and a midwife for a population of several thousand spread along Efate's north coast.

The advantages of rural life for health campaigners are clear. There is a social structure, which provides clear communication channels. More important still, there is a sense of community, allowing village leaders a close familiarity with the people in their area. Even within the Pacific, there is a clear gulf between rural and urban areas. Health workers in Papeete, the capital of Tahiti, were not nearly as familiar with their neighbourhoods as their colleagues in the more rural parts of the French Polynesian island. In the villages, community leaders watched while the people consumed their drugs; in Papeete, they could only hand them out.

AFRICA

Whether they are working in Africa, India or the Pacific, the first step for health campaigners is to meet community leaders. In Africa, this will include village chiefs, church leaders, local councillors and regional assembly representatives. The power of these separate groups varies from village to village, but without key leaders on board, a health campaign is doomed.

In Africa, several tribes have particularly intricate and powerful systems of chiefs. The Akans of Ghana cover 12 separate tribes of which the Ashanti (or Asante) are the most powerful. They make up a pyramid, with a king on top, paramount chiefs below, then divisional chiefs and sub chiefs covering a community of up to three million. The chiefs usually have fulltime jobs, ranging from farming to professional work like law or lecturing. Their positions have sometimes been inherited, but more usually involve appointment by a council of elders. The eldest eligible is no longer an automatic choice and they now have to accede precedence to the most appropriate leader. In the Ashanti, the Queen Mother proposes the more senior appointees, and the elders confirm the nomination. Typically, a council of elders at the village level will have a representative working with the young, another with the elderly, another with responsibility for village development, and another who acts as a health worker. There is usually a women's representative too.

THE CARIBBEAN

In Haiti, there is one other group which health workers have to get on side—the voodoo priests. LF on the Caribbean island is believed by many to be caused by a voodoo curse or an evil spirit—hence the voodoo priest is particularly important in LF health campaigns. It is the voodoo priest to whom many sufferers turn first.

On the map, Leogane does not look far from the Haiti capital of Port Au Prince. It is just 20 miles west along the coast, but the roads are so rutted and eroded, it takes over two hours in a four-wheel drive to complete the journey. What was once France's richest colony is now the poorest country in the Western hemisphere: 8 million people with an average income of $1 a day. Large tracts of what were once verdant hillsides, are now barren land from over-cultivation and the search for wood to provide charcoal for cooking. The former broad boulevards of Leogane, are now pitted with potholes and imposing nineteenth century buildings on either side are dilapidated and crumbling. The island is a desperately sad testimony of the damage which corrupt politics can wreak.

Leogane is a town of 20,000, but its hospital, administered by the Episcopal Church of Haiti, serves a surrounding community of 130,000. About 50% of the population in Leogane is infected by LF and 25% of men suffer from hydrocoele. There are only three tele-

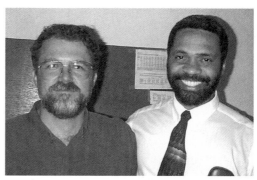

Patrick Lammie at Sainte Croix hospital in Leogane, Haiti with its director Jacques Lafontant.
Source: GSK

phone lines in town—police, hospital and at the telephone company—but frequently all three are out of service. Electricity is only in intermittent supply, although the hospital has an emergency generator. Medics from the U.S. Centers for Disease Control (CDC) in Atlanta set up a clinic within Leogane's hospital over a decade ago. A variety of research and preventive programmes have been run in surrounding villages.

I went with Amanda Freeman, a CDC community worker, to Miton, a village of 350 homes and 2,000 people set among the cane fields and coconut groves outside Leogane. Most villagers were involved with smallscale farming, the women taking the produce—sweet potatoes, casava, cane, corn, mango and bananas—to sell in a nearby market. Every hut had its own charcoal burner. They were grouped in clumps, under the shade of palm and breadfruit trees, separated by cactus hedges. Guinea fowl, hens and bantams were in good supply.

Amanda was a village heroine. A small dynamic blond American, she had built up a wonderful relationship with the villagers and their children. She had helped organise a "mapping exercise" in the village—surveying how much LF the villagers were suffering from—as a first step in an eradication programme. There had been community meetings, a census of every home, an education programme led by the community health worker with 10 volunteers. But the most talked about event was "the filmshow". Villagers had been asked to come to a filmshow at night, when microfilaria would be in their blood. There was no electricity in the village but a portable generator solved that problem. There had been similar video shows before, but never free ones.

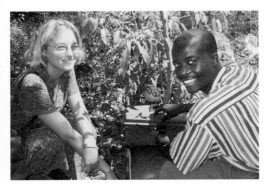

Amanda Freeman and Jean-Marc Brissau with a mosquito trap in Haiti.
Source: GSK

The blood tests were due over three consecutive nights. There were three voodoo priests based in the village, but one lived overseas, another worked outside the village, but the third was crucial. Would he take part in the exercise? The campaigners kept their fingers crossed. If the priest participated, the people would have even

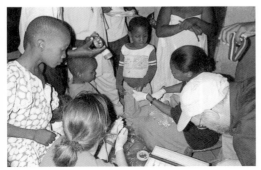

Evening gathering for a night bleed in Leogane, Haiti to test for microfilaria prevalence.
Source: GSK

more faith in the campaign. Two nights passed without any sight of the voodoo practitioner. On the third, just as they had given up hope and were packing up, he turned up and provided blood and urine samples. Subsequent tests showed he was seriously infected. The health team took him to Leogane hospital where, using ultrasound (See Chapter Six), they were able to show him the worms in his lymphatic system. He was converted to the campaign.

I went to talk to the voodoo priest, Charles Barbe, in the temple by his modest home where he conducts his various rituals, sacrifices and ceremonies. A short bearded man, with an open neck white shirt and plain grey trousers, he was suspicious of this reporter, but was reassured by Amanda and her community workers. He said he specialised in leaf treatment, which he had been taught by a voodoo practitioner in Leogane, who had helped put him in touch with the spirits of his Guinean ancestors who had blessed him. He said he treated between 15 and 80 patients a month. He believed diseases could be divided between the natural and the unnatural. The natural should be treated by modern medicine. The unnatural required evocation of ancient African spirits to dispel. He placed LF firmly within the natural category.

AFRICA

Back in Ghana, Margaret Gyapong is convinced the Ghanaian health system has to work out ways of working more closely with soothsayers and traditional healers. They are frequently the first people local villagers turn to and therefore cannot be ignored. Their harmful practises ought to be discouraged and the positive ones encouraged. Margaret worked with her husband, Dr. John Gyapong, the head of research in Ghana's health ministry and coordinator of the LF programme, in the far north of the country for years. (See Chapter Four). Their initial project was a vitamin A programme for 140,000 people that led John Gyapong to develop several LF trials. The north is very different from the south. It is much poorer, surviving on subsistent farming alone. For most of the year it is dry and dusty. Traditionally, the main farming season was compressed into five months, between June and October, the rainy season when the red soil is finally watered. Schools close in this period as the children turn out to help on the land. A major dam on a tributary of the Volta river has allowed dry season projects to spring up along a network of irrigation canals. Farmers have been able to rent adjacent land to grow a wide variety of vegetables—tomatoes, peppers, eggplant and okra.

The villages in the north of Ghana—like the villages in central and northern Nigeria—do not follow a conventional pattern. Far from being a concentrated collection of houses, down either side of a junction of roads, they are spread for miles across the countryside with each family living within a compound of huts, joined and encircled by a mud wall, usually in the centre of the acre of land the family works. It takes a health worker, even with a bicycle, all day just to visit eight households. A typical household has 11 members but some are much bigger. Three generations in one compound are common. There are separate huts for grandparents and children and frequently separate huts for man and wife. The people sleep on mats on the dirt floor. Their main crops are groundnuts, beans, cowpeas, soya and millet. Most meals are vegetarian. The main meal, late morning just before the highest heat of the day, is tuozaafi, a ground millet, with a vegetable soup. The construction of the huts provides a cool resting place in an area where the temperatures regularly climb above 40C.

Out in the field where they work from sunrise to lunch, and then late afternoon to sunset, they eat kuli kuli—a peanut base, which is ground with pepper and spices and then fried. There is milk from goats and the occasional cow, but no meat is eaten except during festival times, when goats and chickens are sacrificed.

There are three tribes, each with their own language, but all with very similar lifestyles. The people of the north, who have far less access to health services, are far more illiterate than the South (as high as 90%). They are much more rooted in ancestor worship and a belief in evil spirits and angry gods. Soothsayers are the first people to whom they turn, not just for health problems but social problems too—money difficulties, family disputes, rows with neighbours.

Soothsayers, who are usually male, offer to get in touch with ancestors for guidance. They call up the spirits through various rituals including a ceremonial spilling of a libation on the earth before passing into trances. They make use of amulets and charms as protection against evil spirits and frequently get paid in kind—two guinea fowl or a bottle of liqueur.

In terms of LF, the people turn to the soothsayers for initial swellings but go to traditional healers herbalists, spiritualists— when the swellings get worse. Margaret Gyapong has seen how close the local people get to soothsayers and traditional healers. She explains: "There are several things we can learn from them. They don't shoo people away. They listen to them. They give them more time than modern medics. They are closer to the people than many modern health workers."

The treatment of traditional healers often do people more harm than good but Margaret Gyapong has been inspired by the way in which Ghana has been able to guide traditional birth attendants towards a more modern midwifery approach. With training in basic hygiene, they no longer cut the umbilical cord with their fingernails and now use special kits, including clean razor blades, to help them deliver babies.

BRAZIL

Margaret Gyapong believes traditional healers are too deeply rooted in local culture for modern health services to be able to divert people from their services. Indeed, it is not just among the illiterate that the culture has such a strong grip. One of the most intelligent LF patients I met in the Brazilian clinic of Gerusa Dreyer (See Chapter Six), was a local teacher who had turned first to a "prayer woman" and then to a "prayer man" for help. She was given the name of the prayer man by her bank manager. Her elephantiasis had developed late and then grown very quickly. Her leg was so large she was having trouble walking and even dressing, because she had lost her sense of balance. She had been told by her family doctor that there was little that could be done for her condition. She explained: "I had no other choice at that time." She spent three days sleeping at the home of a prayer woman. Little turtles were rubbed on her leg, and then special leaves, cooked with herbs, were laid across her legs. Finally, her leg was washed with tea, all to no avail. Indeed, the leaves and herbs, according to Dr. Dreyer, would have encouraged bacteria. In desperation she travelled to a far city, to visit a prayer man.

He prayed with a chicken feather, used a small quantity of seawater three times to wash the leg, re-boiling it each time, and told her she had to believe in his God if she was to be cured. He made signs of the cross on the leg with his eyes shut. But again the treatment failed. She finally found Dr. Dreyer's clinic where, thanks to her modern medical treatment, her leg was already shrinking in size and her acute attacks had stopped.

AFRICA

Traditional healing is not all mumbo jumbo. Some herbal cures do have healing properties. Modern medical scientists in Ghana and East Africa have isolated organic compounds in plants used by traditional healers, and found some close links to modern medicines. But it is much too hit and miss at the moment.

Margaret Gyapong has not given up hope of a better liaison with traditional healers. She has already held several one-to-one meetings with soothsayers and traditional healers in Ghana on how the health service could co-operate with the different alternative services. She found they welcomed the vitamin A project and the LF trials because they were tackling medical problems the soothsayers had been unable to solve. They were still wary, however, of holding a group meeting and worried that modern health programmes might "siphon off their power". This is not going to deter her from keeping open a dialogue and still pursuing her goal of a more formal relationship.

CHAPTER FOUR

The Eradication Challenge

A cursory read of the LF Global Alliance's plans might suggest it had an easy task. What could be easier than an eradication campaign that involves taking just two drugs, in tablet form, once a year for four or five years to ensure the transmission of LF is broken? Unlike the smallpox and polio operations, the LF campaign will not need to organise a "cold chain", involving tons of ice in countries where, in many areas, there is frequently no electricity. The LF drugs are far less sensitive to heat than the smallpox and polio vaccines. They come sealed in small cartons, with instructions to keep the containers tightly closed, protected from light, in a dry place and below 30C (85F). Stability tests have shown that albendazole retains its full potency for up to five years after the cartons have been opened and the seal broken; Mectizan for up to 12 months.

Unlike the West African OCP river blindness programme, which was closely linked to massive insecticide drives on the river breeding sites of the blackfly which spreads the disease, LF will succeed with just drugs. It is planning to link up with anti-mosquito programmes—like bed nets—but will be effective without these programmes.

A third advantage which LF faces compared to preventive programmes such as Guinea Worm, is that it is not trying to change human behaviour. Changing human behaviour can be the most challenging of tasks, requiring people to change habits of a lifetime. A key part of the Guinea Worm campaign is teaching villagers to filter all their water through special nylon cloth before drinking it. Guinea worm is transmitted when people consume drinking water contaminated by tiny water fleas carrying the larvae of the Guinea Worm (*dracunculus,* which gives the disease its medical name: *dracunculiasis*). Inside the body, the larvae penetrate the intestinal wall and develop into a threadlike worm up to three feet long. After about a year, the worms emerge through painful blisters on the skin. The campaign has persuaded sufferers not to rush into ponds or streams to cool the blister because that is how the female worm discharges her larvae, which then infect the fleas and restart the cycle.

Smallpox and polio involve viruses but no vector—such as a mosquito or other blood sucking insects. There are a large number of vector borne diseases including malaria, LF and dengue (all mosquito borne), sleeping sickness (tsetse), Chagas (kissing bug). No vector borne disease has yet been eliminated. Guinea Worm looks set to become the first, and, if the LF campaign succeeds, it will be the second.

Clearly the LF Global Alliance enjoys certain advantages over earlier campaigns, but as noted in the opening chapter, it also faces steeper challenges. The first is that local people were much more aware of the threats that smallpox and polio posed. Everyone knew someone who had had these diseases. The devastation they caused was all too apparent. One fifth of the smallpox victims died—and the other four suffered immense pain and ended up with badly scarred faces and bodies. They could not be missed. The paralysis which polio inflicted was known to villagers too. They were familiar with the funerals that frequently followed. LF is not a fatal disease, but is grossly disabling and disfiguring. Much of it is unseen. Only 10% develop elephantiasis, which can't be hidden. Hydrocoele has much bigger numbers but hugely enlarged scrotums can be hidden. Kidney and lymphatic damage is totally invisible. Moreover, LF cannot be eliminated with one vaccine jab. It will need four to five years of dual drug doses. Politicians were eager to get involved with the polio campaign. LF's lower profile generates less political involvement yet the campaign needs far more public education than earlier campaigns.

The second major challenge is the numbers who will have to be treated. Smallpox began as a mass immunisation programme, but quickly became a targeted campaign. Polio is only vaccinating the under fives. LF is having to treat not just the 120 million infected but the 1 billion at risk. To put that in perspective: when the widely-admired 14-year-old river blindness Mectizan Donation Programme reaches its peak, it will be treating 50 million people a year.

How do you persuade people who are not sick to take the tablets? That is where the benefits of albendazole come into play—albendazole's capacity to kill five separate intestinal worms. Wherever I have watched the distribution of the drug, there have been eager takers. Even illiterate peasants are aware of the devastating effects that intestinal worms have on their own nutrition—and even more important on their children's physical and intellectual development. One West Indian survey showed a single treatment for a single worm, whip worm, produced a dramatic improvement in learning.

Children may not be aware of the effects of worms, but they are aware of the effects of tablets and the dead worms they subsequently pass. One small boy in a school-based Haitian programme I visited, could not get over the size of the dead worm. He raced up to the health workers, eyes wide open, describing the length of the dead worm with the index finger of each hand, rather like an excited fisherman after a big catch. Parents whose children had been in earlier trials told me about how their children were growing faster and taller since being dewormed. They were also less anaemic and sleeping better, making them more energetic and more able to benefit from school. They were only too eager for their children to take part in the eradication campaign, recognising how the disease was a financial catastrophe for families as well as a personal tragedy for children.

Pilot LF programmes in India had no trouble in attracting the uninfected as well as the infected. The grapevine had told the villagers just how much better hair looked after a dose of ivermectin. It also drastically reduces itching.

These additional health benefits have not just helped promote the programme but also resolved the serious ethical issue
facing the campaign. How can it justify giving drugs to people
who are not ill? It is now not only able to point to earlier immunisation programmes which have done just the same, but it can
also show clear and important health benefits for the uninfected
as well as the infected.

A third challenge has been attracting the support of affluent
donor countries. LF has long been eradicated from affluent tropical states. Unlike smallpox, it poses no threat to these affluent
states. Moreover it is not a fatal disease, just a seriously disabling
one. There has been less incentive for the affluent to get involved.
The GSK and Merck donations transformed this problem but has
not resolved a more fundamental issue: the reduction in health
spending across much of the developing world.

A succession of reports from WHO and the World Bank has
warned of the danger of the squeeze on health spending in general
and preventive health programmes in particular. Preventive health
programmes have been suffering even more seriously than hospitals and acute services. Effective prevention achieves far bigger
health and economic gains than acute treatment. Immunisation
saves the lives of an estimated three million children a year. Better
control of diarrhoea saves another million. Yet international and
national cuts to health budgets have continued. A 1995 World
Bank survey of 53 states found a 15% decline in health spending.
Emergency aid rose in 1998 while health care funding continued
to drop. The OECD group of affluent states reduced their funding
to poorer states in 1999 to the lowest level since 1991.

WHO's 1996 World Health Report spoke of the hundreds of
millions of people in low and middle income countries on the
threshold of an era in which they will be safe from some of the
world's most threatening diseases. In its 1996 report on the State
of the World's Children, UNICEF showed the proportion dying
before the age of five was less than half the level of 1960. The 1997
annual WHO review reminded the world that increased longevity
without quality of life was an empty prize—"health expectancy is

more important than life expectancy"—but welcomed the reduction in disability among older people in some populations. The 1998 review, marking WHO's 50th anniversary, remained cautiously optimistic that "longer life can be a prize worth winning". Major infectious diseases—polio, Guinea Worm, river blindness, leprosy, Chagas—were "steadily being defeated".

A WHO report in June, 1999, noted the world was in danger of missing its chance to eradicate some of the biggest killer diseases, including TB, malaria and AIDS, which were becoming resistant to drugs and spreading through foreign travel. Just six killers (AIDS, malaria, TB, measles, diarrhoeal diseases and respiratory diseases such as pneumonia) accounted for 90% of all deaths from infectious diseases among people under 44. Gro Harlem Brundtland, WHO director general, described the report as "a wake-up call to the world's governments, decision-makers and private sector to take action before it is too late."

The West still reacts well to natural disasters like earthquakes in Turkey, floods in Venezuela and cyclones in India. But as a report from the International Federation of Red Cross and Crescent Societies noted in June, 2000, the death toll from infectious diseases is 160 times greater than the number killed in natural disasters. It went on: "Unfortunately, infectious diseases create silent disasters, which often go unrecognised and unreported. Unlike the 'sudden strike' events such as hurricanes and earthquakes, they fail to attract the media spotlight or trigger the flow of donor dollars into primary health care."

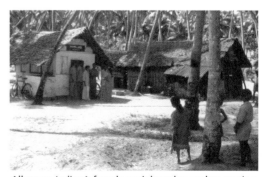

Alleppey, India: A female social worker on her routine visit to one of the volunteer clubs in a rural area.
Source: WHO/TDR/Chandran

Many states in which the LF campaign is being launched have been hit by the reduction in overseas aid and a reduction in internal revenue for health under various debt and economic reconstruction programmes. Some are spending less than $10 per person on all healthcare in a year. Most are spending less than $20. Yet these same health ministries are also involved in fighting malaria, AIDS, respiratory diseases, serious diarrhoea, TB as well as more exotic vector-borne tropical diseases like schistosomiasis, onchocerciasis (river blindness), and dracunculiasis (Guinea Worm).

The economic benefits of eradication programmes are clear and unequivocal. In India—where one third of all LF cases occur—the disease costs almost $1 billion a year in lost production. Male weavers with chronic LF in India have an estimated 27% lower productivity than colleagues without the disease. In sub-Saharan Africa, men with hydrocoele lose between 20% and 60% of their productivity. As many as 40 million men could have hydrocoele in the region. LF's economic burden in the region has been estimated at $1.7 billion each year—83% of the loss due to the disabilities of men with hydrocoele.

It is not just the direct costs of lost productivity from the chronic and acute conditions. There are the add-on costs of patients seeking treatment. About 10 million LF sufferers seek treatment in India every year. Millions more should be seeking help but don't in the mistaken belief there is nothing that can be done. In northern parts of Ghana, where LF is particularly endemic, health officials estimate about 25% of all operations are for hydrocoele repair. A 1995 study in China documented the benefits which eradication achieves. Three academics carried out a cost-benefit analysis of eliminating LF in a township of Huzhou City in Zhejiang province and concluded that every $1 invested in LF control produced more than $15 in economic benefit. A World Bank study of the Guinea Worm programme in Africa showed a 29% rate of return on investment in the eradication programme.

These separate studies on the costs of LF in China, India and Africa only underline the importance of the World Bank's conversion to investment in health, particularly given that it has a budget of $11 billion a year compared to WHO's $1 billion. Its 1980 policy paper announcing the Bank's decision to begin lending to health programmes, was particularly concerned with infectious diseases and malnutrition because they accounted "for the majority of deaths among the poorest people in poor countries." But in a 1997 report on Health, Nutrition and Population, the Bank acknowledged the continuing damaging economic impact of non-fatal but disabling diseases. It noted the long term and irreversible retardation of physical and mental health that can occur. It also recognised how good health added to the overall quality of life as well as to productivity. In the new jargon, rather than just extending life expectancy, campaigners should be aiming to prolong health expectancy.

Much more needs to be done as the 1997 WHO report on the progress of the control of tropical diseases reported. It noted the response of the international donor community to disease control had been inadequate for many years. But it went on: ". . . in recent months there has been renewed interest by the donor community as the economic, social and political impact of the disease burden on developing countries has become more evident." It heralded the new agreement between GSK and WHO on the elimination of LF that promised to accelerate economic growth, improve living standards, and raise education levels for 1.2 billion people living in endemic countries. It added: "This agreement will not only have an impact on the well-being of one fifth of the world population, but also represents a new class of global cooperation in health. Hopefully it would set a precedent for many such arrangements in years to come."

Beneath the current financial squeeze, there is a more fundamental problem: an ambivalence among health workers about eradication programmes. Part of this ambivalence has been fed by the failure of earlier eradication programmes. The Rockefeller Foundation's hookworm elimination project in 1907 reduced the severity of the individual infections, but rarely eradicated them which led to rapid reinfection. Undaunted, the Foundation tried to eliminate yellow fever in 1915, but failed because of the unknown cycle of the disease among monkeys and apes in the forests. Following the failure of these campaigns, eradication

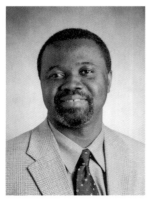

Source: GSK

DR. JOHN GYAPONG
An African Public Health Pioneer

There was not much career guidance in secondary schools, even for clever pupils, when John Gyapong was at school in Ghana. If you were good at science, you were told you would be an engineer or a doctor. If you were good at arts, you became a lawyer. John Gyapong was good at science. His father was a nurse in the military services. He was sent to medical school in Kumasi, capital of Ashanti land, one of only two medical schools at that time. It was in the early 1980s, tempestuous times. The people were in revolt against a corrupt civilian government. As a student leader (head of a hall of 500 students), young John felt torn: "There was a genuine revolutionary feeling. The country was in terrible trouble. We felt we should not be in academia but helping the nation."

His dilemma was resolved. The universities were shut down. Student leader Gyapong led a group to the main port servicing Accra, where they spent several months unloading cocoa. But he finally got back to medical school and has been able to help his nation in all manner of pioneering public health programmes since.

It began in his first year after graduation from medical school. He heard of a massive vitamin A supplement trial starting in the far north of the country, close to the Burkina Faso border, that required a paediatrician to help run the programme and monitor the effects on children. It was a dry, dusty and impoverished region with no electricity, phones or regular piped water but he signed on for a year and got caught by the public health bug. "It dawned on me that most of the problems we saw in the clinics could be reduced by good public health programmes."

After one year, he extended his contract for the other two years of the programme. For a young graduate, it was an amazing programme to be running: 140,000 people spread across a massive area with every household involved. It was in his second year that he began studying LF too. He was working in Ghana's most endemic region and was seeing a high incidence of elephantiasis, lymphoedema and hydrocoele. "As we were visiting every family to check on vitamin A and nutrition, it was not difficult to add LF." Thus began his long association with the North and LF—and not just himself but his wife, Margaret, a medical anthropologist, too.

His research earned him a Masters at the London School of Tropical Medicine and Hygiene in 1992 and four years later a Ph. D. (Few of the lecturers, let alone a graduate student, had run such a huge trial.) He dashed back to Ghana, between his two degrees, to set up a new research project into LF after winning a prestigious WHO grant ear-marked for the disease. All his earlier research projects have helped him in developing Ghana's current LF programme. His dissertations were on designing interventions for LF and looking at the social and economic impact of the disease. Another early research project involved devising an easier and cheaper way of mapping the disease, rather than using conventional blood tests. It also demonstrated that lay (non medical) interviewers could be trained to inquire and obtain a very accurate map of the disease. This was done by carrying out a survey of the prevalence of hydrocoeles in 30 communities in three different districts. In his words: "An eradication campaign does not need to know who is infected, but which communities are infected."

His other research work includes a dual drug trial on 12,000 patients; and a comparative exercise checking the effectiveness of two different ways of distributing drugs (See this chapter). His wife is equally indefatigable. Margaret recently organised a monitoring exercise in which 130 compounds, ranging in size from six people to 150, were visited every 14 days to chart the development of LF in every person in the household for an entire year.

Like many Ghanaians I met, Johnny Gyapong is a gentle, humourous and committed public servant. Although a serious researcher, there is nothing solemn about the Ghanaian way of life. It still finds time for fun and laughter. But the commitment is serious. He was the perfect man to be put in charge of the LF programme: well organised, imaginative and ready to try new approaches. If only there were more of him. Only six out of the 32 medical students in his graduation class are still working in Ghana.

went out of fashion in the 1920s and 1930s but emerged again in the 1940s with the elimination of the *Anopheles gambiae* mosquito in Brazil and Egypt and the reduction of yaws in Haiti. In 1955, WHO launched eradication campaigns against malaria and yaws, which failed according to the 1993 International Task Force report, partly because latent cases were not treated adequately.

Even the success of WHO's smallpox campaign in 1977 failed to remove all scepticism of eradication programmes. Halfdan Mahler, WHO's third director general, who launched the much needed drive to improve primary health care in the late 1970s, was one sceptic. He suggested: "Important lessons can be learned from smallpox eradication but the idea that we should single out other diseases for worldwide eradication is not among them."

D.A.Henderson, the leader of WHO's eradication campaign against smallpox, has noted how narrowly victory was achieved: "As I look back, I realise that had the biological and epidemiological characteristics of the disease, or the world political situation been slightly more negative, the effort would have failed."

The continuing ambivalence of some health workers was well described by the report of the Dahlem workshop on "The Eradication of Infectious Diseases", edited by Walter Dowdle and Don Hopkins in 1997: "Many individuals, both national and international, struggling to improve health with limited resources see eradication as a detour around their own priorities; their path of resistance is that 'the task is impossible' and that the resources should not be wasted on an impossible task. Others see the political and/or technical barriers as insurmountable."

I met Walter Dowdle, former deputy director of the massive U.S. federal government's CDC and then head of the Taskforce for Child Survival in his Atlanta office. A small, compact and wise man, he speaks very softly. He was deeply involved in the smallpox and polio campaigns, but understands the opposition that eradication programmes still raise. They could divert resources and even contradict the aim of integrated primary health care systems. That was why eradication programmes should be constructed to help strengthen primary health care—through, for example, training programmes for community health workers that had a wider application.

He went on: "Many people in the developed world find it difficult to think there could be resistance to internationally subsidised health programmes in developing countries. They need to place themselves into African shoes. Practically every little village out there has had some helicoptered scientist fly in and fly out pretty quickly. It builds up a certain degree of cynicism. There is goodwill in these communities but there is also considerable suspicion of drug companies, scientists and public health officials from the developed world. One of the biggest challenges of the Alliance will be to find a common ground on which trust with local communities can be built."

He ticked off the advantages of eradication programmes: internationally it was easier to sell single measurable interventions than a primary health care doctrine of integrated services; not only were the interventions visible but they carried a presumption of a successful finale; primary health care had no end, but eradication programmes had clear end goals. One problem of community health programmes was a tendency to become too curative focused, as noted in the WHO report on smallpox, rather than giving preventative health programmes their due priority.

Then there were the two big advantages set out by the International Task Force for Disease Eradication in 1993: First that eradication is permanent, as are its benefits. In contrast, the costs of control programmes continue indefinitely, along with the risks of future exacerbation of the disease following a disaster of natural or human origin. For some diseases, achieving control would require only marginally less effort than that needed to achieve eradication, but control measures would need to be continued indefinitely. Eradication was the ultimate "sustainable" improvement in public health. Second, a time-limited goal of eradication allows mobilisation of support for a concentrated effort more readily than does a control programme—both within countries where the disease is endemic and internationally.

Over at the Carter Center, set in beautiful grounds on the other side of Atlanta, Don Hopkins, who helped set up the International Task Force and has been steeped in public health campaigns was even more succinct about what an eradication campaign can do for a community: "The lives of these people will be forever affected by eradication. They will know they can change things. Their lives will improve. They will say 'What else around here can we change'. Whole countries will grow stronger."

Back in Geneva, Eric Ottesen, WHO coordinator of the LF elimination programme, is fully aware of this debate. He is more familiar with the plans for national LF eradication programmes than anyone else, as all the state applications to join the LF Global Alliance have passed across his desk. He insists: "This eradication campaign will strengthen the health infrastructure. It will stretch it in the way that exercises help stretch and strengthen athletic performances. It will not only deliver long term benefits in eradication of LF, but also provide lessons on how to mobilise support within communities, which will be of direct benefit to a much wider group of diseases and health problems."

It needs to be added that the success of the current polio and Guinea Worm campaigns have only widened support for eradication programmes. I watched Dr. Gro Harlem Brundtland, WHO director general, launch the final push against polio in January 1999 in India. A disease which once infected millions was then down to 7,000. The Indian subcontinent, which accounts for 70% of the total, is well equipped to eliminate their last cases. Africa will find it more difficult. Even so, Dr. Brundtland pointed to the progress. When the WHO campaign began 12 years ago, 1,000 children a day were being paralysed by polio; by 1999 this was down to 30. The last push began in a poor part of east Delhi, where 100 young sari-clad mothers, forming a colourful waiting rainbow, had brought their infants for two drops of oral vaccine from a small plastic vial. Dr. Brundtland, surrounded by television cameras, began the new round of immunisation. The previous year 470 million children worldwide—two-thirds of all children under five—were immunised in the campaign.

The LF campaign re-opened another old health debate: should it be a vertical or horizontal programme. Smallpox, polio and river blindness all began as vertical programmes—organised from the capital of the particular country with immunisation teams moving from one community to the next. Both smallpox and polio, as explained above, changed strategy to a more targeted approach, but most health specialists still categorise the new approach as vertically driven. But about halfway into the 14-year-old river blindness campaign, the organisers switched to a horizontal approach, extending much more discretion to community delivered programmes. (See Chapter Five).

William Foege believes the debate poses a false dichotomy. He discovered the debate was going on as long ago as 1886 in the US, when its health infrastructure was like the developing world's today, far from comprehensive: "It forced me to think what had happened over 100 years ago in America. When we had something that worked, we tried to deliver it. Infrastructure was developed by doing one thing after another that worked. Don't let us waste time going round the argument. We should be delivering what we can. The big problem today is that we are getting more and more things that we can deliver so they start competing. We have to be cautious and wise how we deliver things. We must ensure programmes we have started, like the eradication of polio, get finished. The LF campaigners should be asking all the time: how do we do this in a way that improves the infrastructure."

Some of the earliest LF Global Alliance programmes have been in the Pacific. It was an appropriate region for such early campaigns. In no other region of the world has the disease been studied more seriously. American, British, French and Japanese scientists—as well as indigenous doctors—have all worked on the disease in the region. Few states have had such extensive experience of earlier drug administration programmes. The tiny island nations, with strong social structures still in place in rural areas, have a long history of battling with the disabling disease. They are also familiar with the biggest challenge facing eradication programmes—the need to keep going, even when infection has dropped to two per cent or less, to ensure eradication.

Some 22 Pacific nations, comprising 1,000 islands and seven million people, have come together under the umbrella of PacELF (Pacific elimination of lymphatic filariasis). About 350,000 people are infected by the disease, but all seven million are at risk. Supported by WHO and initially funded by aid from Australia, PacELF is now primarily funded by the Japanese government. It aims to rid their region of LF by 2005 and achieve a formal declaration of elimination by 2010—10 years ahead of the global goal. The three small island nations of Samoa, American Samoa and Niue launched programmes in 1999. I visited Vanuatu for the launch of its programme in June 2000, and then went to Tahiti (French Polynesia), to discover its post launch lessons.

There is no single approach, even within one nation, but Vanuatu is a good illustration of the challenge. As described in Chapter Three, Vanuatu is a Y-shaped archipelago of 83 tropical islands, 64 of which are inhabited, just south of the Solomon Islands, about a two-hour flight from Australia or New Zealand. Over 75% of the 200,000 population live in rural communities, their first and prime loyalty being to their village, not their island, let alone the nation of 83 islands. By the nature of this society, health campaigns have to be decentralised.

I watched an all day seminar in Port Vila, the attractive national capital, to which 40 key community health workers from the 14 islands in the Shefa province had been invited. The 20 males sat down one side of a large rectangle of tables, and another 20 colourfully dressed women down the other—community nurses, midwives, health centre managers, dispensary supervisors, health promotion workers, and malaria, TB and leprosy campaigners. Half were French speaking, half English. Several village chiefs were included in their ranks.

George Taleo, an impressive and dynamic national organiser, set out the framework: the drugs that would be distributed to each village; the literature to help health workers and volunteers; the registration books in which the dosages which patients

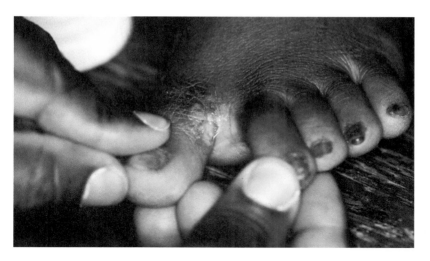

Damaged and infected skin in between the toes is a prime entry point for secondary infections of the leg.

Source: WHO/TDR/Crump

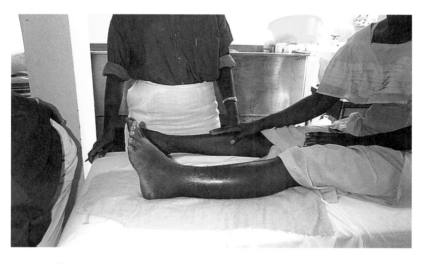

Young Haitian woman experiencing an acute attack of limb swelling and fever.

Source: GSK

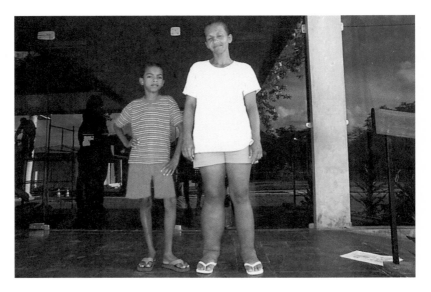

Brazilian woman with lymphoedema.
Source: GSK

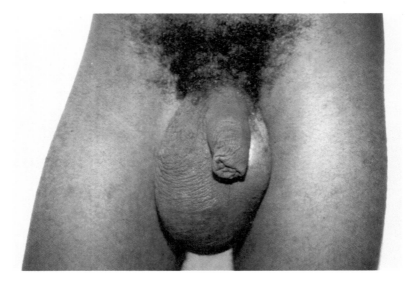

Unilateral hydrocoele.
Source: T Streit, Notre Dame University

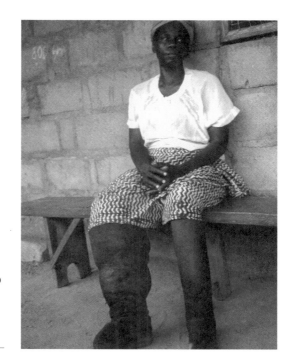

A Ghanaian mother of two sits showing elephantiasis of the right leg and oedema in the left.
Source: WHO/TDR/Crump

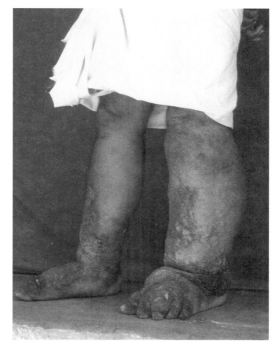

Indian male with elephantiasis of the legs.
Source: WHO/TDR/Chandran

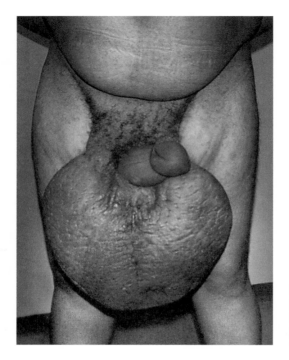

Brazilian man with
elephantiasis of
the scrotum.
Source: GSK

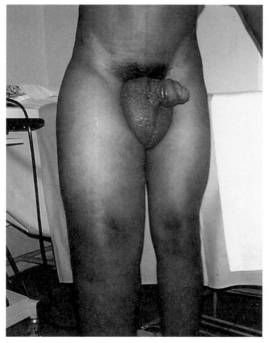

Brazil: 14 year old boy
with hydrocoele and
lymphoedema.
Source: GSK

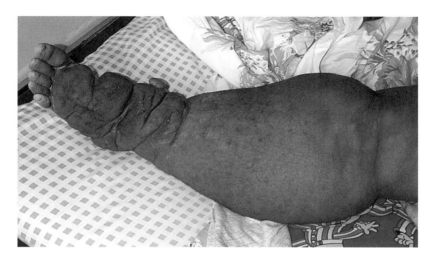

Brazilian woman with elephantiasis and deep skin fissures.
Source: GSK

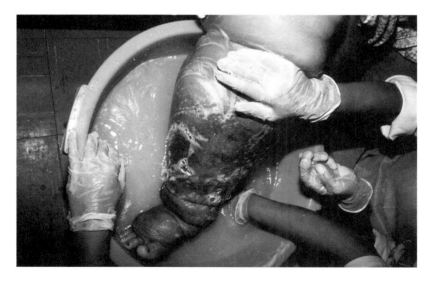

Washing the legs of a Brazilian woman with elephantiasis.
Source: WHO/TDR/Crump

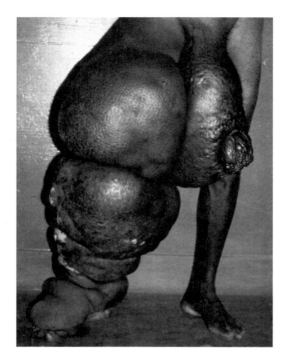

Chronic elephantiasis of right upper and lower limb as well as scrotum and penis in a 50-year-old Indian male.

Source: WHO/TDR/Ramachandran

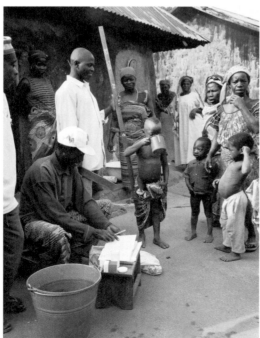

Togo: Boy swallowing tablets at a village distribution.

Source: GSK

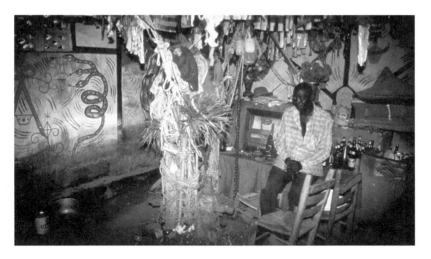

Leogane: A 60-year-old voodoo priest, who has oedema of the right leg.
Source: WHO/TDR/Crump

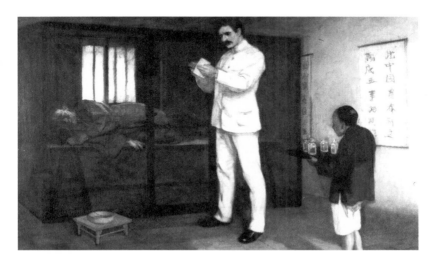

Sir Patrick Manson depicted observing human LF infection by mosquitoes.
Source: Wellcome Trust Library

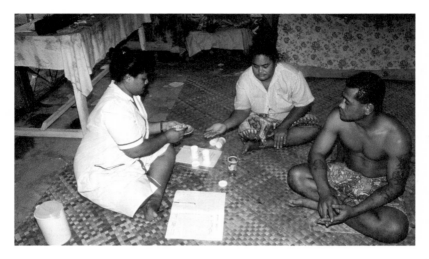

Community distribution of albendazole and DEC on Monono Island, Samoa.
Source: WHO/TDR/Crump

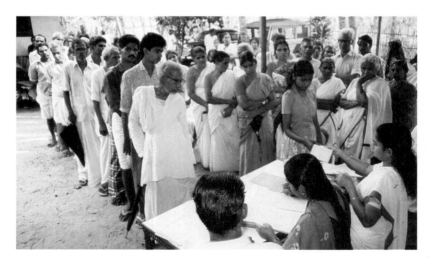

Patients, including many young children, lining up for registration at the Filariasis
Clinic, Vector Control Research Centre VCRC in India.
Source: WHO/TDR/Chandran

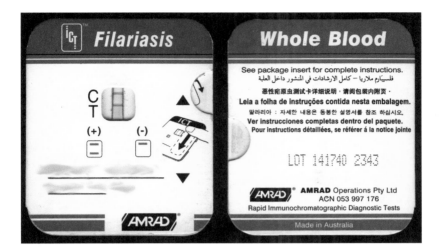

ICT Card Test for Filariasis.
Source: GSK

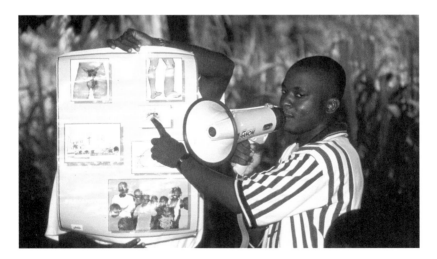

Health workers in Haiti inform the community about the disease.
Source: WHO/TDR/Crump

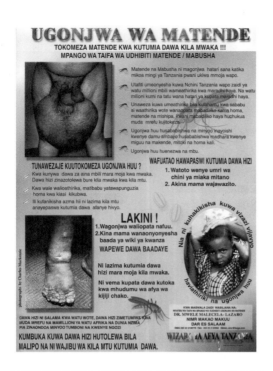

Tanzania LF educational campaign poster.
Source: Tanzania National Institute for Medical Research

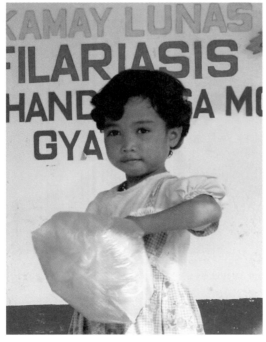

"Filaria Fair" in the Philippines.
Source: GSK

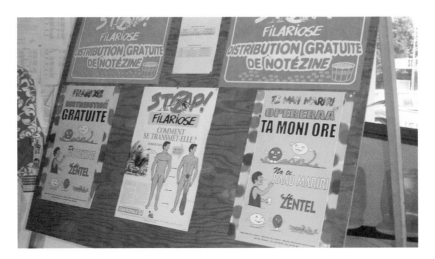

LF posters in French Polynesia.
Source: GSK

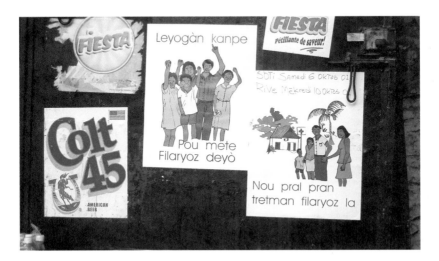

LF posters in Haiti
Source: GSK

A Pharaoh's Affliction

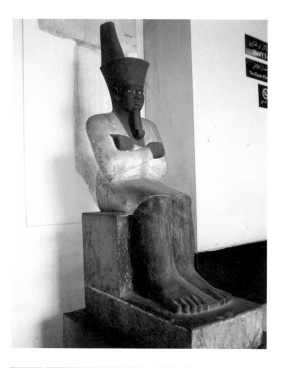

Cairo Museum: Statue of an Egyptian Pharaoh depicting possible signs of elephantiasis.
Source: GSK

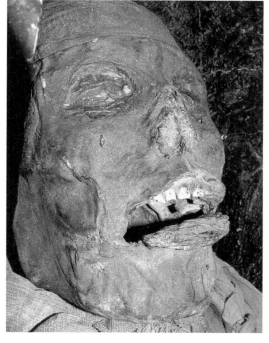

The mummified body of Natsef-Amun, a priest at Karnak in the time of Rameses XI (1113–1085 B.C.) proven after 3,000 years by autopsy to have LF worms in the groin.
Source: Leeds Museum

received would be registered; the different doses of DEC (according to height and weight) which patients should receive, along with the standard white tablet of albendazole which all would receive; and the national mobilisation campaign (radio, local press, television on the few islands with access, posters and pamphlets) which local campaigns could link into. There was a local radio and TV reporter present for much of the day, to add to the public education programme. He even took his tablets on camera to encourage the islands.

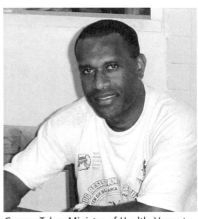

George Taleo, Ministry of Health, Vanuatu.
Source: GSK

The framework was clear but key decisions on how the dual drugs should be distributed was left to community workers. Some planned house-to-house visits by local health teams; several others decided to distribute from a community centre. They argued it would allow village chiefs, local church leaders and health workers to be more involved. Even on the main island, four-wheel drive vehicles are needed to negotiate the frequently flooded coastal road. On other islands, access to some communities can only be done by boat. On others, internal communities can only be reached by foot. (On one French Polynesia island, the health team followed the delivery vehicle of the main store, handing out the drugs to people turning out for their provisions. They achieved comprehensive coverage.)

Before the launch of the LF Global Alliance in 1998, few people were worrying about LF in Vanuatu. The launch prompted an epidemiological survey across Vanuatu's islands. Health officials thought LF was only infecting certain islands. They were wrong. The survey covered 5,000 people from 51 villages. Only one island was found to be LF free. Several others had low infection rates, but in the most endemic areas, 50% of people were infected. This was followed by a public education programme, which was in full swing when I arrived. Even local theatre groups had been enrolled to produce campaign awareness raising jingles for community radio stations. Vanuatu, which as a colony was jointly run by the British and French, has had a succession of governments and has numerous political parties—cynics suggest one for each of the 64 inhabited islands. But the LF campaign coincided with a more stable government, which was only too ready to back the campaign and win some kudos.

On hand at the Port Vila seminar was Kazuyo Ichimori, WHO regional coordinator of the elimination programme. A tiny but indefatigable character, she played an important behind-the-scenes role in the creation of PacELF. Typically, when invited to speak at the Vanuatu seminar, she gave only the briefest of speeches although she had been steeped in the preparation of the campaign. Sensibly she left it to local health officials to run the day. A WHO regional post is no place for a big ego or big heads. PacELF may have raised the money (initially from AusAID and then Japan) for the crucial support costs that are needed to supplement the free drugs in the LF project, but national programmes will only succeed if they feel a sense of "ownership".

The Pacific may seem like a single community to outsiders but there are three distinct cultures—Melanesian, Micronesian and Polynesian—with many sub cultures. It needs adroit diplomatic skills and subtlety to move within these 22 nations encouraging take-up of the LF campaign, but not breaking cultural rules. Trained in Japan and the U.S. with field experience in Africa and Central America, Ichimori had the best possible preparation.

How is a nation like Samoa, never colonised and sturdily independent, encouraged to take part? It leaped at the chance of leading the world, its Prime Minister taking the two drugs on television, its famously successful rugby team following suit, and even the British, French and U.S. ambassadors invited to parliament to take the drugs and maintain the mobilisation campaign. Samoa believes it has achieved 96% coverage of its population in 1999 and 2000. Tonga, which is more traditional, required a different approach.

French Polynesia had completed its first annual 2-drug treatment programme when I got there in June 2000. A nation of five archipelagos totalling 130 islands (88 inhabited) spread across an area the size of Europe, this was no easy task. Yet the success of the campaign in the more rural areas, where villagers took the two drugs in front of health officials, was easier to assess than urban Papeete, the Tahitian town that is the nation's capital. Almost half of French Polynesia's 200,000 people live in or around Papeete. There was a high profile campaign in the capital using radio, TV and posters. The health minister took his pills

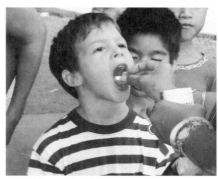

School-based distribution in French Polynesia.
Source: GSK

on television. For school children, there was a filariasis week during which the drugs were distributed. For adults, there was an LF day. Everywhere one turned in the capital, a stall was manned by health workers and volunteers, handing out the drugs—supermarkets, pharmacies, health facilities and the massive covered market, to which most locals turn, in the centre of the town.

Those that missed out on the day could still obtain the free drugs for a week from health facilities. About 95% of the necessary tablets were distributed but Lam Nguyen, a highly intelligent epidemiologist working in the nation's main research unit in Tahiti for the last 11 years, drew a distinction between distribution and coverage. The pills had been distributed but the campaigners felt unable in the urban area to require people to take them in front of health workers. Life in the city is too busy. They did not want to deter people, who did not have the time to consume the drugs and have their dose registered. In an earlier era of French central control, people were threatened with fines if they did not take their drugs. That authoritarianism is no longer realistic.

Lam is aware from his research of a familiar pattern in disease control in the Pacific. Twice in the past 50 years, French Polynesia believed it had eliminated LF as a public health risk only to see it re-emerge. In the 1950s, up to 40% of the population on some islands were infected. The introduction of DEC in 1953 cut the prevalence in 15 districts from 30% to 3% by 1959, only for it to begin to climb again when officials moved from active to a passive programme. A similar pattern occurred in the 1980s. This third campaign will benefit from the failures of the previous two drug administration programmes and the much more powerful effect of the drug combination. Ichimori, for one, is determined that it will be third time lucky in French Polynesia.

The smallpox campaigners wanted an early—and challenging—target where they could demonstrate success and built momentum for their programme. They went to West Africa where they were supremely successful. The LF Global Alliance is also looking at West Africa and has selected Ghana to lead the way in the LF campaign. Just over one third of the country—the top northern third plus the coastal area in the south—has been mapped. An outstanding researcher, Dr. John Gyapong, has been made programme coordinator for Ghana's LF campaign. He is acting director of the national health research unit at the Ghana Ministry of Health and is extremely familiar with the disease. It was Dr. Gyapong who was selected to report on the African scene at the London conference in January, 2000, when the formal strategy for the elimination of LF was unveiled in Manson House, the home of the Royal Society of Tropical Medicine. Later in the year in Santiago de Compostela in northern Spain, he reported on African developments at the first meeting of the LF Global Alliance.

Dr. Gyapong has answered a crucial operational question with research into the most effective means of distributing drugs. This involved 40 villages, each with 1,000 people, spread across four districts. One half had their drugs delivered by the health service. In the other half, the health service left it to the community to decide how the drugs should be collected and distributed. The second proved far more effective in getting drugs to people. Typically, in better organised areas, a district (140,000 people) will be divided into five sub districts. Each sub district would have a health centre and a team of up to 10 health workers to serve a population of 27,000. Following Dr. Gyapong's research, Ghana will be placing considerable emphasis on community-directed treatment (CDT) in its LF programme for rural areas. Dr. Gyapong explains: "The health system does not have enough people to go into communities and deliver drugs. My research found them using all sorts of excuses, such as no petrol or no vehicles, but the main problem is shortage of staff. It is easier to use one health worker to link up with 10 communities to set up a community-directed treatment programme, than to say to the health worker they are required to distribute this large batch of free drugs to 1,000 people in 10 communities. As long as you set up a system with proper documentation and training, we have demonstrated the drugs will be delivered. CDT programmes select volunteers who can read and write and are familiar with figures."

In urban areas, the approach will be more vertical with a well-publicised immunisation day in which LF drugs will be handed out from a variety of points. People who miss out will be able to get their free drugs from health facilities for a numbers of days that follow. LF will not be the first community-based programme in Ghana. The Guinea Worm campaign began as a community-based programme in 1989 and has seen the number of cases fall from 180,000 to fewer than 6,000 and the number of infected villages decline from 6,500 to 650. That is one example of the effectiveness of community based programmes.

Encouraged by the LF Global Alliance, the different health campaign leaders—LF, Guinea Worm, river blindness—are all talking with each other and examining ways in which they could co-ordinate their activities. They are also talking with the new campaign team against trachoma, the eye infection that leads to eyelashes turning inwards, scarring the cornea and leading to blindness. Pilot coordinated campaigns are being planned for Nigeria (See Chapter Five), Ghana, Tanzania and Togo.

Asked whether Ghana's pilot LF programme had found difficulties in persuading people without the disease to take the drugs,

Dr. Gyapong declared: "Not at all. It is not as difficult as it might seem. Our earlier disease control programmes have helped build up trust. Our education programmes have ensured that the people are aware of the additional benefits—the intestinal worms that will be killed, the scabies that will be cured, and the lice eliminated. It does not take the bush telegraph long to communicate how much better most people feel once they have had the drugs."

CHAPTER FIVE

Dual Campaigns—
The Piggy Back Option

Another idyllic scene—another country. Deep in the heart of Nigeria, we reached a small river that had been partly dammed by a crude bridge crossing it. The bridge had created a natural swimming pool on one side and a bubbling waterway on the other. A small gang of exuberant naked children were having a glorious time, jumping into the water from a sandy bank. There was even a shallow end for smaller children, complete with a sandy beach. Beyond the beach there was a lush green landscape. It was early July, one month into Nigeria's rainy season. All adults and older children were in the fields, weeding their millet crops.

"Isn't that wonderful," I said to my companions, only to be contradicted by one of my guides, Dr. Frank Richards, the technical adviser based in Atlanta of the Carter Center's river blindness (onchocerciasis) campaign. With a rueful grin, he explained: "That scene incorporates three crucial health threats to these people: a fresh water pool in which water snails, which can harbour the schistosomiasis larvae, will get a ready supply from children with the bilharzia disease urinating in the water; fast running water on the other side, where the black fly which spreads onchocerciasis can breed in the well oxygenated water; and the calmer waters below, provide a breeding ground for mosquitoes that will spread LF."

Frank Richards is no pessimist. He knows the only way of surviving in public health is optimism. He has all the energy and intelligence of my other companion, Abel Eigege, a gentle Nigerian

63

pharmacist, who is the Carter Center's assistant national director for LF and schistosomiasis control. They are key players in a trial which hopefully will show that all three diseases—LF, oncho and schistosomiasis ('schisto', or bilharzia)—can be tackled in one integrated programme. We had driven for over two hours across the hot red plain of the Plateau State, and then another hour along a rutted ill-defined track through lightly wooded hills. It was cooler in this upper part of the state that was so verdant and green; it felt like England until the occasional flame tree, or baobab (water trees) or mud and thatch settlement hoved into sight.

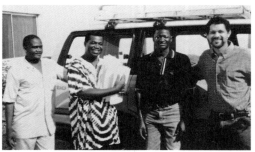

(L-R) Lliya Haruna, Abel Eigege, Bitrus Sule and Frank Richards in Jos, Nigeria.
Source: The Carter Center

The track wound its way through a succession of "villages"— like northern Ghana, the villages are not concentrated collections of houses, but are spread out for miles with each household having its own compound of mud huts, each with a conical thatched roof, joined together by an outer mud wall. Typically, there are eight huts in a cluster, but chiefs have more than 12—separate huts for separate wives, children, livestock and granaries. Frequently, just outside the compound, is a smaller thatched hut and pen—a house for the family pig and its piglets. The families farm the surrounding acre of land and frequently rent larger plots further away.

We were heading for Mudel, a village of 140 households and 1,000 people to launch the first piggyback trial. This was the culmination of two years work involving officials and medics from local, state and federal government; the Carter Center's staff at its field centre in Jos, the pleasant capital of Plateau State; and LF Global Alliance team members in Geneva and the US. It could not be more crucial to the success of the LF campaign. Almost from the launch of the Alliance, the search has been on for ways in which LF can link up with other health programmes. For obvious reasons: governments at all levels—federal, state and local—do not want to set up special structures for an exercise that only involves taking two drugs, at the same time, on one day of the year. The aim is to coordinate—and integrate—LF with other appropriate programmes.

The one obvious programme for such integration in Africa is the river blindness campaign. There are already two separate and well-established programmes in operation fighting this disease. The OCP (Onchocerciasis Control Programme) was launched in 1974 in West Africa. Initially incorporating seven countries, it was expanded to 11 in 1986, and now covers 30 million people. The OCP is due to wind down in 2002, when it is expected to have prevented 600,000 cases of blindness and added five million years of productive labour to the economies of its member states. At its launch one million people in the area were suffering from the disease, of whom 100,000 had serious eye problems and 35,000 were blind. By the mid 1990s, the number of infected people within the original operations area was, in WHO's assessment, "practically nil".

The main thrust of OCP was the use of selected insecticides that were spread by aircraft on the main breeding sites of the black fly in fast flowing rivers. Once the cycle of river blindness has been interrupted for 14 years, the reservoir of adult worms dies out in the human population. By 1995, the parasite reservoir of the original seven states had virtually died out and elimination was expected in the other four by 2002. For the last 14 years, OCP member states have been offered free ivermectin (Mectizan®), under the Mectizan Donation Programme organised by Merck & Co., Inc. The drug, when provided as a single annual oral dose, kills the disease's microfilariae, helping to save the sight of hundreds of thousands.

In June 1994, the World Bank (which coordinated the international donors of the OCP programme) launched a new initiative, the African Programme for Onchocerciasis Control (APOC) which has introduced a river blindness control programme in the other 19 African countries, outside OCP, where the disease remains. These countries have had generous donations from the Mectizan programme. By April 1996, the programme was eight years old and had delivered 50 million treatments. Two years later, this cumulative total had reached 100 million treatments. In 2001 they will achieve 200 million.

Nigeria has the biggest oncho programmes. In 1999 there were more than 13 million treatments for the disease—4.5 million, or 34% of the total assisted by the Carter Center's Global 2000 River Blindness Programme (GRBP) that operates in nine of Nigeria's 36 states. The campaign was initiated under the River Blindness Foundation (RBF) in 1991, in collaboration with the Nigerian Ministry of Health, and absorbed into the Carter Center's GRBP project in 1996.

There is one obvious reason why 'oncho' campaigners could become suitable partners with LF campaigners: they are both using the same ivermectin drug in Africa. Oncho only required ivermectin, but the addition of albendazole (again as a single oral dose) adds effectiveness against LF, without reducing ivermectin's effects on oncho's microfilariae. But there are other reasons too. The oncho programme has already established a structure, down which the drugs flow from federal, through state and local government to the village level, and the people's mouths.

Structures are in place to provide the other crucial services needed for a successful health campaign: health educators to mobilise take-up and organise public posters, radio plugs and other publicity; a political network with contacts at local, state and federal level to draw in political and civil service leaders behind the campaign; extensive training courses for village health workers, community drug distributors, and their managers. Frequently, village health workers are unfamiliar with the causes and transmission cycles of diseases, which they need to know before they talk to their communities, as well as the more practical organisational needs of an eradication programme. The Carter Center alone helped to train 15,000 community drug distributors and village health workers last year, plus almost 500 managers at its headquarters in Jos, and in its regional outposts.

The Carter Center in collaboration with the Federal Ministry of Health is co-ordinating the current trial, testing the viability of the three prong campaign against LF, oncho, and schistosomiasis. It has approached it in its normal thorough and impressively professional manner. The aim is to conduct the trial in two states—Plateau and Nasarawa—which were trial states for the River Blindness Foundation's oncho programme in 1992. The aim is to produce a model that can be used across Nigeria. Of the three diseases, only oncho has been thoroughly mapped in Nigeria. But there was a rough survey by the national coordinator for LF and schisto, Dr. M.Y. Jinadu. She wrote to all newly graduated doctors, who have to spend part of their first year in rural areas, asking them to report on the diseases in their areas. This showed LF was endemic in 32 states and schisto in all 36. This could be an underestimate for LF. Wherever the LF team has conducted a mapping exercise, even in areas where it was not expecting it, infection has been found. LF campaigners believe it will be found in all 36 states.

The trial scheme in Plateau and Nasarawa began with a mapping exercise in two separate local government areas, which were known to be endemic for oncho. Detailed surveys for LF and schisto were carried out in 230 villages. Individual medical histories were taken down, physical examinations for scrotal hydrocoele carried out, and antigen blood tests conducted. Only seven out of 152 villages were found to be LF free. Infection rates in the rest ranged from 3% to 67%. There was a mean prevalence of 24%. Only six out of 180 villages were found to be schisto free, with infection rates in the rest ranging from 3% to 73% with a mean prevalence of 20%.

While this was being conducted, an equally important knowledge, attitude and practice (KAP) survey in six villages was being conducted to test attitudes in local communities towards the two new diseases being added to oncho control and their knowledge of them. There were focus group discussions, semi-structured interviews and lists of diseases which people were asked to rank in order of importance. Care was taken to ensure there was equal representations of males and females, as well as a representative cross section of all generations, from young to old.

Dr. Eigege, who was in charge of the LF/schisto operations, found there was widespread awareness of the diseases but also widespread misconceptions of their causes—a familiar cause of hydrocoele being put down to adultery while the blood, which schisto produces in the urine, was seen as a rite of passage to adulthood or male menstruation. The people were grateful for the oncho programme and positive about the planned expansion to a combined drug strategy. It was clear from interviews with infected people, that they would continue to use both traditional healers as well as modern medicine. This is one reason why Dr. Eigege is exploring ways that traditional healers could, with training, be brought into the programme.

The KAP programme provided a fact file around which health education material was produced—posters, brochures, flip charts for community drug distributors, and a thousand copies of a calendar with educational information on schisto, all of which were tested in two villages selected as pilot programmes.

The LF Global Alliance's safety review of combining albendazole and ivermectin delayed a possible starting date for a triple trial. Nigeria opted instead to proceed with its oncho programme and introduce a separate schisto trial. Unlike the oncho and LF programmes, there is no long-term promise of free drugs for schisto. Worse still, the wonder drug for this disease, praziquantel, costs 40 U.S. cents per patient, which is expensive in states that spend only $10 in total per person for all health needs. But thanks to limited drug donations from drug companies that produce praziquantel (Bayer Pharmaceutical of Germany, Medochemie of Cyprus and Shin Poong of South Korea) plus a financial donation from GSK, the Carter Center was able to run a programme for 50,000 people between October 1999 and October 2000.

The programme covered 102 villages. Virtually all were oncho and LF endemic as well. Some 23 villages, where there was high schisto prevalence, had mass treatment. Another 79 villages treated only the most vulnerable age group, children aged five to

14. Community drug distributors first treated children in school and later tracked down the 20% who were not in school. Impact studies showed there were immediate effects with people no longer passing blood in their urine within two to three days. In 2001, 100 villages will be treated for all three diseases—LF, oncho and schisto.

With the dual albendazole and ivermectin doses cleared by the safety review, Nigeria had one last hurdle to pass before the world's first trial of a dual oncho/LF campaign could be launched. Under the safety procedures of the LF campaign, agreed to in Geneva, every national LF programme has to conduct small-scale safety trials to check for adverse results. Nigeria chose two small farming communities in Plateau state for the April 2000 trial—the village of Kadyis, where prevalence surveys suggested 57% of the population were infected with LF and Nyelleng, a slightly bigger village with 40% LF prevalence. Both had been dosing people with ivermectin for seven years under the oncho programme. Each village received an extensive health education programme explaining all three diseases.

The plan had been to treat 2,000 people with the dual drugs but the programme ended up treating all 2,252 people in the two villages who turned out. There was little reluctance to come for treatment in either village. They were already aware of the side benefits of ivermectin in terms of controlling lice and scabies and, to a lesser extent, worms. The bush telegraph—as well as the education programmes—told them how much more effective albendazole would be in killing worms. With many of the villagers not wearing shoes, hookworm was a problem, and round worms were even more common. Each village was treated on the same day by separate teams, each led by a doctor.

For the first four days after treatment, two physicians and seven community health officials were resident in the two villages. For the following three days, one physician and the seven health workers were present. They saw, recorded and gave basic health care to all people reporting adverse effects. Patient monitoring forms were filled out and sent back to Geneva. The Nigerian teams found the highest incidence of reporting reactions was on day one (treatment day) to day three. Even so, only 5.6% reported any reactions over seven days. The other 94.4% were free of any adverse effects, prompting the teams to speculate whether combined dual drug doses ameliorate ivermectin's single dose adverse effects.

Adverse effects were divided into three categories: mild, moderate and severe. There were no severe (defined as completely interrupting daily activities) and only 11 people with moderate effects (some interuption of daily activities), most commonly headaches, which did interfere with work by requiring people to lie down for two to three hours. Other effects included abdominal, joint and muscle pains, but none were long lasting. Of the 108 people with mild reactions, the most common complaint was a headache but 41 suffered some abdominal pain, 34 pain in their joints, 20 dizziness and 19 some fatigue, but none needed to take any time off work.

What the monitors also received before the end of the first week were warm thanks from the villagers for getting rid of their worms. The villagers had had no difficulty in identifying the large dead round worms that passed out with their stool within 24 hours of taking the drugs.

Dr. Eigege was euphoric. Back at the Carter Center's field station in Jos, a delightful hill town used by missionaries in their heyday, the Carter campaigner explained: "It was better than our best hopes and gave us the all-clear to start the campaign proper."

Thus it was that I found myself travelling with Drs. Richards and Eigege on the way to Mudel, the first village selected by the Nigerians to start the world's first integrated programme to tackle LF and oncho. There are 100,000 villages in Nigeria. There are 7,000 villages in the two states of Plateau and neighbouring Nasarawa alone. The Mudel villagers knew it was lucky. Health educators had been in to explain. But they were not aware just how lucky they were, although the arrival of a white foreign reporter in a four-wheel drive vehicle told them something very special was taking place.

The villagers were assembled at their traditional meeting place, a large locust bean tree, with huge spreading boughs providing shade. The villagers boil the beans and make a sweet pudding from the powder in the pod. The tree was just to the side of the sandy track. About 400 people had been waiting earlier for the great event, but we were late, and so many had moved back to their fields to continue weeding their millet. About 200 drifted back on news of our arrival, women collecting on one side of the tree, men on the other. There were friendly smiles, much laughter and an eagerness to talk—particularly, with the help of interpreters, to the foreign white reporter.

The villagers are virtually self-sustaining—with flour from millet and maize, plenty of fruit (mango, guava and banana), egg and meat (pork, goat and chickens). They consume half their cereal crops and sell the other half for their small cash needs—kerosene for lamps, salt, palm oil for cooking, soap and clothes. Many lived in three generation households. One old man, in what in the West would have been called a grandfather's collarless shirt, had turned out for his drug dose. Aged 80, he was one of many who had been born, brought up and still lived in the village.

There was only one well in the village—and that was only six years old. The women placed an extra well at the top of their wish list. Some had a daily two-hour journey—one hour each way—fetching water to their homes. A stream runs through the village all year but village health workers, too, were anxious for a second well.

Just near to the tree trunk, stood a small wooden desk, a chair, and a stick with height markings cut into its bark. On the desk were three registration books and white cartons filled with albendazole and ivermectin. Every member of all 148 households had been set down in the registration books. There were columns for their ages and the size of their dose. Albendazole has a standard dose for all, but ivermectin is dependent on weight or height. The biggest farmers needed four tablets. Children under five, pregnant women, breast-feeding women and the sick were all excluded and marked in the books as U (under age), P (pregnant) or S (sick). Health details used to be kept on cards kept in each family compound, but as some families tended to lose them, the programme switched to registration books kept by health workers, not families.

Sani Jugu, a public health official from the Plateau ministry of health, described to the villagers what was going to happen. A health education programme had already been run in the village. It was not long before they were asked to line up. The chief, with his four wives, headed the queue, then the men, finally the women and children. Each had their height measured, were handed the pills, and a blue plastic mug of water. Most could swallow with the smallest of sips. The children were told they could bite, or suck the albendazole tablet, which had been sweetened on purpose to make it more palatable. Dr. Richards and myself ate one too, to reassure the children they tasted good. The various details were logged by one of three community health workers. Their job, when all 200 had been logged, was to track down the other 700 villagers spread across the extended village, to ensure they took their drugs.

The programme is by no means problem free. The biggest problem is the cash shortage. Everyone I met—health workers, community workers, local and state officials—spoke of transport problems. There was not even enough cash for bicycles to help in the distribution of drugs. A motorcycle was regarded as the ultimate luxury. Four-wheel drive vehicles were reserved for foreign reporters.

The dual programme desperately needs more money. Frank Richards spoke of the need to "leverage" the generous GSK support to obtain new grants from other international donors. The Gates Foundation grant has begun this process. Phase Two, which begins in 2001, aims to treat 650,000 people across the two states. Phase Three, the following year, aims to reach two million. Phase Four hopes to reach all four million in the two states. This will be a much wider population than the oncho programme, which runs mostly along fast-flowing rivers.

Oncho itself has its problems. The Carter Center in its regular reports openly talks of the shortfall in funding, the irregular release of approved funds, delays in state and local council budget-making processes, the wide variation in contributions made by villagers to community drug distributors, delays in village registration, not to mention occasional communal clashes which had historically disrupted public health programmes.

In his Jos office, I met the state commissioner for health, Dr. Dabiyak Damulak, who was equally frank about the dire financial position. He had moved in with the new civilian government as the military government moved out. One of the last acts of the military in Plateau was to sell off the health ministry's three working vehicles, leaving Dr. Damulak with two unworkable ones and the commissioner's car. There were only two computers in his entire office and no printer.

But there is a more serious oncho problem, which could affect LF. Dr. Emmanuel Miri, the gentle and widely-respected head of the Carter programme in Nigeria, is resolute about the need for a wider debate. The current approach to distributing ivermectin for onchocerciasis under APOC is called CDTI—community-directed treatment with ivermectin. The aim is an unambiguously worthy one: to move public health administration even closer to the people it helps. The shift to a much more locally administered service has resulted in the need for all training to be carried out at village level. This is more cumbersome and time-consuming but clearly manageable. More serious is the discretion now extended to communities to decide when their treatment programmes should begin. The LF program needs simultaneous treatments if LF transmission is to be interrupted. Dr. Miri was issuing warnings of the dangers that an uncoordinated approach by the two programs in a state of 7,000 villages would produce disaster.

Dr. Miri is also worried by the lack of supervision and monitoring in the new system. Human administration, he suggests, is not as sharp or conscientious if it knows it is not going to be audited from outside. He worries the community based workers won't follow up families, who have not taken drugs, as diligently if they are being monitored. It may be unpopular in a devolution age, but he argues that "you get better coverage and better results if it is centrally directed".

Frank Richards has raised another issue for APOC. In a letter published in the *Lancet* in 2000, he noted that APOC's ivermectin distribution strategy is only designed to control onchoceriasis eye and skin disease, but not halt transmission. The onchocerciasis program only provides ivermectin in villages where the prevalence of infection is over 20%, a strategy which will not prevent new infections from occurring.

A joint LF/oncho programme could help to resolve this issue. The LF campaign requires treatment in villages with as low an infection rate as 1%. This may ensure that villages with oncho infections of less than 20% may now be brought into the new joint programme. A separate problem is that the current stretch of the programme will have to be considerably extended. LF is believed by many health workers to extend over an area at least three times as large as oncho. This will be a major challenge.

Back in Jos, at a conference for Carter Center assisted health programmes in Nigeria, a delegate asked a most appropriate question: "Now we have EPI (expanded programme on immunisation), isn't it time for an EDA (expanded drug administration programmes)?" The answer was short and simple: "Yes it is time and the proof is it can be done. We've got one with the joint oncho/LF programme and the three pronged oncho/LF/schisto project."

CHAPTER SIX

Helping the Afflicted

There were about 60 people in the main theatre of Pernambuco University in Recife on the northeast coast of Brazil. Suddenly they erupted with joy, rushing forward to greet a small neatly dressed woman on her arrival. Small handmade gifts were thrust into her hands. There were hugs, kisses and applause. These were people whom for years had been told there was "no treatment" and "no hope". All 60 were suffering from LF.

Dr. Gerusa Dreyer, who in her early days at the university's medical school, Brazil's oldest, had been given the same message but refused to accept it, has proved her former professors wrong. Not only has she given patients hope—the patients were all attending Recife's "New Hope" club—but after long and often lonely years of research, with many parallels to Patrick Manson's pioneering work identifying the cause of LF over 100 years earlier, she's demonstrated that what was thought to be untreatable is treatable. Better still, the LF treatment does not require expensively-trained medics, but can be carried out by the people themselves. Even better, it does not require expensive equipment or drugs, but basic nineteenth century rules of hygiene including washing, simple skin care, the elevation of affected limbs at night—and where possible in the day, too. Together, these simple procedures not only can halt the progression of the disease, but may even reverse it.

Proof of her success could be found on virtually every occupied seat in the theatre. One older woman there, whose condition had become so severe she could not even get off her bed, is back running her home and looking after three of her 10 grandchildren. Another woman, a former teacher, whose leg had grown so large she found it difficult to dress herself or maintain her balance while walking, was now an active organiser of the club and a strong advocate of the LF eradication campaign.

The hope club began a decade ago with the aim of providing LF patients with the skills, motivation and enthusiasm that would sustain their low-cost, self-care treatment. The club has been so successful it now has four branches—separate sections for patients with lymphoedema, hydrocoele, chyluria (patients

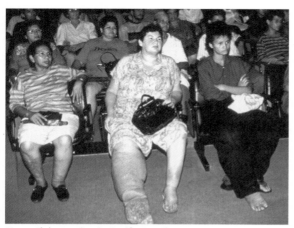

Hope Club meeting in Recife, Brazil.
Source: WHO/TDR/Crump

whose urine contains leaked lymph fluid turning it white) and a fourth for child sufferers. The support which they give each other is all too apparent. So is the sense of optimism and empowerment. Here was a powerful group of patients, who recognised they were not on their own. Just a few months earlier, when drought had reduced Recife's clean water supplies, it was the patients who organised community "foot washing centres" to ensure their daily hygiene routines were not interrupted.

Above all else, however, was a sense of fun. Several new patients were at the meeting I attended. Out came a series of cartoon slides, with a series of questions on how they should wash their affected arms and legs: where do germs party? (Between the toes and in skin folds). Which doors do germs use to enter the body? (Cuts and lesions). Should blisters be pricked? (No.) This part was conducted by Patricia, Gerusa's dynamic daughter, now in her fourth year at medical school. Answers were chanted back by the happy crowd. And there was even more fun in a competition to find a new name for soap. "Gerusa the germ chaser" won.

Earlier in the day I had climbed up to the fifth floor of a central hospital block, where between urology and infectious diseases, Gerusa sees her patients. Special foot baths have been built plus a ward with three beds. Although the emphasis is on simple procedures, some complicated work is done. A handsome young man, who turned up with his attractive fiancee at the hope club, had had his scrotum reconstructed.

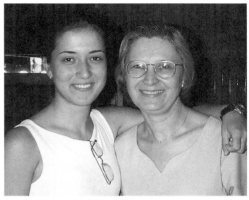

Gerusa Dreyer (right) with daughter Patricia Dreyer.
Source: GSK

One key to Gerusa's success as a researcher is her clinical work. Eric Ottesen, who went to see her in her early days, explains: "LF is not an easy disease to work with as a researcher because there is no laboratory model. Mice and rats are no help. Humans are the only host. You have to find your patients and work with them. Gerusa has a wonderful relationship with her patients. They were starved of hope and medical attention and then they found her. She gave them hope and personal medical attention and they gave her access to the disease. She has a probing, questioning mind and is an astute medical observer."

The six patients I met in the clinic could not have been more different. A mentally handicapped teenaged boy with elephantiasis of both legs, and hydrocoele; a wild teenaged girl, who had been threatened with amputation of her swollen leg, now well on her way to recovery; an athletic 28-year-old anxious businessman; a serious middle-aged teacher; and a 29-year-old woman with lymphoedema of the right leg. The saddest case was a 31-year-old man, who worked as a meat supplier. His lymph nodes were wrongly removed as a child, prompting a leak of lymph fluid from his scrotum. He had to wear sanitary towels to keep himself dry. When these got too wet, the fluid burned his skin. Intercourse with his wife had almost stopped, both because of the leakage and the awful odour of the fluid.

Gerusa's medical success story begins in her fourth year at Pernambuco. It was there that she met her first elephantiasis patient. The patient's main concern was not with her own condition but whether there was some way her new grandchild could be protected from the disease. Even so, the fourth year student asked her professor whether anything could be done for the patient. She was told there was nothing. An eradication campaign might help the grandchildren but the grandmother's condition was untreatable.

Undaunted, Gerusa refused to accept the advice. Until then, as the oldest child and first to go to university in a family of immigrants—her mother being German and her father, Romanian—her plan had been to pursue a high-tech highly paid medical career in order to help her three younger siblings through university, too. She still managed to help with the latter goal through various second medical posts, but her determination to discover some effective medical relief for LF patients, meant there was no chance of earning lucrative private fees. Indeed, in the last 15 years, she has at several points shared her modest public salary with younger colleagues in pursuit of her research goals.

While still a student she read as much as she could about the disease and the related disciplines needed to conquer it—immunology, parasitology, pathology, urogenital medicine and surgery. Shortly after her graduation, the Brazilian state research institute, the Oswaldo Cruz Foundation (Fiocruz), decided to set up a five-member research unit in tropical medicine in Recife. She was invited to be a member but was told she could not pursue LF; she would have to concentrate on malaria. Undeterred, she proceeded to pursue her LF research at night which, given the nocturnal nature of the disease's microfilaria, she would in any case have been required to do. She went out late, collecting blood samples from local communities, to identify patients and track the pattern of the disease. She was twice robbed returning from late blood-collecting trips but resolutely continued with her research.

Indeed, she took on an extra teaching load to help her cover early research costs—syringes, needles, lab tests.

Another two years later, Fiocruz allowed her to switch to LF. She continued to teach, to explore new morbidity control techniques with her growing number of patients, and to pursue a wide range of research. By 1988 she had a group of 1500 men, 93% of whom had infection in the scrotal area, whom she has continued to track ever since. She persuaded the Brazilian armed services to allow her to screen their recruits in the region, which added another 25,000 case histories between 1988–92 to the 10,000 already in her own database. This database now numbers 43,000.

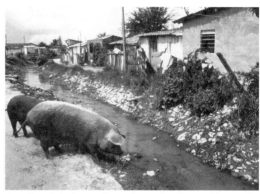

A polluted drainage channel at a favela outside Recife, Brazil makes an ideal site for mosquito breeding.
Source: WTO/TDR/Crump

Dr. Dreyer's first break came through Eric Ottesen to whom she sent a series of specimens from her patients. She is engagingly frank about their first meeting: "I wanted to meet him. I could see the humanity behind his massive research. But when I learned he was coming to Brazil, I was in a panic. I had taught myself about the disease through the literature. I did not know how to pronounce the words, or even his name. My spoken English is not good." She need not have worried. Dr. Ottesen recognised her quality straight away.

Dr. Dreyer's rejection of the conventional theory of the time—that the swellings which LF caused was something to do with the LF worm and its disruption of the body's immune system—was prompted by a basic medical instinct: "There was something wrong with the idea that a bad odour could be caused by a worm." She went back to first principles: hygiene. As early as 1986, she decided to test whether it was bacteria entering through lesions that was the main cause of the problems. She noticed that patients with damaged lymphatic vessels or lymphoedema frequently had more bacteria on the skin than usual. They were either unable or did not know how to wash properly. They frequently had small cuts, or scratches in the skin, or between the toes. It was through these "entry lesions" that bacteria could be entering the body and multiplying quickly.

She decided to wash the legs of the patients herself, finding it difficult to convince them that it would help. But it did. Almost immediately. Her first patient slept through the night for the first time for years after having had her legs properly washed. She enrolled 600 patients in this experiment and continued it for six years before publication. She wanted to be totally convinced about the results. By the end of six years she was.

Patients were given meticulous step-by-step lessons on washing: soaping with room temperature water, beginning at the highest point of the swelling, usually the knee, then washing down to the feet. Those with severe swellings, who found it difficult to reach their limbs or toes, were encouraged to get children or grandchildren to help. They were taught to examine their limbs for entry lesions, to wash them well, dry carefully, and where washing did not heal them, to use a variety of antiseptic, antifungal or antibacterial agents.

Her research suggests 97% of acute attacks are caused by bacteria entering through lesions in the skin, not by the LF worm. The worms account for only 3%. By persuading her patients to follow a systematic approach to hygiene, skin care, elevation of affected limbs and simple exercises of affected feet or limbs, she was able to achieve a reduction in the swellings of between 50% and 90%, depending on the severity of the case.

She taught her techniques during the 1990s to Jacky Louis Charles, an engaging and enthusiastic Haitian physiotherapist, working at a CDC-supported clinic at the Hopital Sainte Croix in Leogane, a coastal town with the highest prevalence of LF in Haiti. Jacky trained in North America before going out to Dr. Dreyer's clinic in Recife. He began his clinic in Haiti in 1995, and has achieved similar success rates to Dr. Dreyer. He now has a data base of 600 patients. Like Dr. Dreyer, Jacky teaches his patients how to wash and dry their limbs and search for lesions, particularly between their toes and in the folds of their swollen limbs. Home visits are organised so patients can be advised on the best approach in their domestic setting.

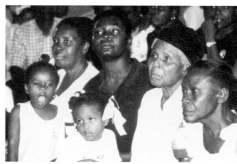

Hope Club Meeting in Leogane, Haiti.
Source: WTO/TDR/Crump

Like Dr. Dreyer's patients, Jacky's patients too are full of spirit, fight and gratitude to the clinic for the relief it has produced. I went on a tour with Jacky to his patients in Leogane, in what was once a prosperous provincial town with wide tree-lined avenues but now, like much of Haiti, is rundown and dilapidated. There are only three working telephones left—at the hospital, police station, and the telephone company—in the town, and even these are frequently not operating. The missionary hospital, which serves a population of 130,000 people, struggles along with outdated equipment, shortage of drugs and trained staff, yet it has helped pioneer and prove Dr. Dreyer's regime.

At the entrance to the hospital is a patient with a particularly poignant story. Antoine Maurice, who has large soulful eyes, sits by the gate selling soft iced drinks to patients, many of whom have travelled for miles. He was one of Jacky's first patients, deliberately sought out by the physiotherapist. Jacky had remembered seeing Antoine's huge legs as a boy. Antoine was employed by a local distillery, driving big containers of sugar cane syrup to the rum factory on an ox cart. As a boy, Jacky was scared by Antoine's swollen legs and the danger of becoming infected. Once trained, he knew Antoine did not pose any risk and could be helped if he could be tracked down. He was. Although the disease had reached its most severe form—stage seven in which decomposing parts of the leg come away in the hand—he was taught how to wash himself, provided with loose stockings to protect his legs from flies, and given specially made sandals to fit his swollen feet and protect them from further cuts. The legs are still large but the swelling has been reduced; his skin has regained its suppleness; the knobs and cauliflower surface and odour has disappeared; and he no longer suffers from acute attacks.

Meanwhile, another dedicated CDC researcher with a base in Haiti, Dr. David Addiss, joined forces with Gerusa Dreyer in producing separate handbooks—already translated into five languages—for patients and health workers round the world. The pamphlet for patients, "New Hope for People with Lymphoedema", sets out in a series of cheery illustrations how patients should practice good hygiene and the different ways they can elevate their limbs—pillows under the end of a mattress, legs on a stool at meal times, or even when feeding babies or working at a desk.

Quite independent of Recife, health workers in two other parts of the world—in Tanzania and in Alleppey in India—were following a similar line to Dr. Dreyer's. Eric Ottesen explains: "Gerusa is not the only researcher to have identified bacteria as the key agent in the development of elephantiasis, but she has carried this research further than anyone else and gone on to develop the correct clinical response to controlling morbidity."

WHO, with the support of the Japanese government, commissioned Gerusa along with David Addiss to run a series of international workshops to train leading health workers round the world in her approach. Using the training manual they produced in March 2000, the two researchers will guide community health trainers through six learning units—on community treatment, the lymphatic system, the assessment of lymphoedema, the management of the lymphoedema, the assessment and management of acute attacks, and urogenital problems including hydrocoele.

If Dr. Dreyer's research had been restricted to the influence of external bacteria entering the body through lesions, she would have made a significant mark. But her research ranges far wider than this. She has developed a new diagnostic tool—ultrasound— that has not only identified damage to the lymphatic system at a much earlier age than previously believed, but has given researchers new means of measuring the progress of the disease, the effects of drugs on the condition, and the number of nematode (worm) nests in a patient's lymphatic system. She has participated in pioneering surgery, which not only removed the first live worms from the lymphatic system (the male was named Eric), but which also validated the ultrasound diagnosis. And she has redefined the disease, bringing to much more prominence, the high incidence of hydrocoeles in more than 50% of infected men.

It took Dr. Dreyer four years of badgering her medical colleagues before she persuaded a sonographer to test whether patients without any apparent symptoms of the disease could already be infected with worms. She became fascinated by patients without symptoms: "I felt sure they were still suffering from the hidden disease. My colleagues said I was crazy and told me to go away. Finally, I persuaded a sonographer to look at an asymptomatic male. The ultrasound identified a nest of worms. The sonographer said it must be an artifact, but I sent another 14 patients without symptoms, seven of whom turned out to have worms."

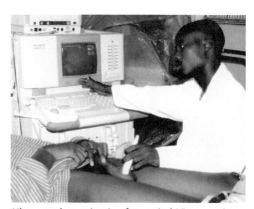

Ultrasound examination for genital LF worms in a male at Hospital Sainte Croix, Leogane, Haiti.
Source: T Streit, Notre Dame University

Her research—some 80 published papers in total—has achieved a breakthrough as important for the afflicted as Sir Patrick Manson's original research was for public health officials intent on eradication. There are close parallels between the two researchers: both have worked as clinicians in isolated units, were cut off from the main research centres, and are mainly self taught. To their credit, leading researchers in the main centres—like Eric Ottesen and David Addiss—embraced her work and have helped promote her new clinical methods.

CHAPTER SEVEN

Building an Alliance

Appropriately, it was a famous and historic pilgrimage city, Santiago de Compostela in Northern Spain, that demonstrated the LF Global Alliance was alive and well and ready to fly. In early May, 2000, just one million albendazole tablets had been shipped. Two months later, eight million had been shipped and by the end of the year 34 million.

Over 70 representatives from 30 partners were present in Santiago in May for the inaugural conference of the LF Global Alliance. Just as the early pilgrims traditionally joined forces to provide mutual aid in the face of the many challenges on their journey, so modern day public health campaigners create coalitions for a similar purpose.

There was no doubting the success of the Alliance's architects looking round at the Spanish conference. Just 27 months following the January 1998 joint announcement by WHO and GSK, an impressive alliance was in place. All the necessary interests in public health were represented, although ideally even more partners and bilateral donors were still needed. The three key international organisations had signed up as partners: the World Bank, the United Nations Children's Fund (UNICEF), and WHO; three private sector firms: Merck & Co. Inc., the American pharmaceutical company with a key drug, AMRAD ICT, an Australian company manufacturing blood-testing antigen cards at a cost price to map the disease, and GSK; eight international development agencies or foundations from Australia, Belgium, Italy, Japan, the Netherlands, Spain, the U.K., the U.S. and the Arab Fund for Economic and Social Development; and eight major non-governmental organisations were lending support, among them the Carter Center in the U.S.; Health and Development International, Norway; Interchurch Medical Assistance, U.S.; the Centre for Partnerships in Health, Australia; and the World Alliance for Community Health, Canada (See full list at end of chapter).

All these were backed up by 10 academic and research institutes based in nine different countries. These included the world's leading tropical disease institutions: the Centers for Disease Control in Atlanta; Emory University in Atlanta; and the Liverpool School of Tropical Medicine, U.K..

It would be wrong to assume that the path from the heady announcement in January 1998 to the inaugural conference in May 2000 was as smooth as the old stone alleyways in ancient Santiago. The 27 months involved considerable sweat, blood and tears from the team that WHO and GSK had set up to create the Alliance. But achieve it they did.

There were 27 months of working parties, task forces, research initiatives and conferences before the ship sailed into Santiago. The subject areas were infinite ranging from the fundamental structure of the programme to the most detailed examination of how countries should be adjudged ready to join the programme. All manner of questions had to be answered: was the 20-year target date too short for a campaign that required people at risk to take five annual drug doses, rather than a single vaccination? Or was it too long, given the difficulty of maintaining campaigns beyond 10 years? The solution was a 20-year campaign with four phases. On one issue there was no debate: the need to expand the partnership widening the campaign beyond WHO and GSK.

Even before the two bodies announced their pioneering collaboration, WHO had been talking with the World Bank, the Arab Fund for Economic and Social Development, and the Centers for Disease Control in the US. The need for a global alliance was apparent to all. Indeed, there were genuine fears that the WHO/GSK announcement might prompt key international players in disease control, whose expertise and support was urgently needed, feeling left out. Both WHO and GSK officials moved quickly to dispel any feelings that other partners were not wanted.

The world has moved on since smallpox days. The smallpox campaign, which was directed by WHO, was driven by the U.S. which provided most of the specialists in the early days and much of the money. In the initial campaign, in West and Central Africa, it even provided free measles vaccine as well as the smallpox vaccine. But the U.S. is no longer ready to be as benevolent. Its overseas aid budget has been drastically reduced by an inward-looking Congress. And international aid has moved on with bilateral donors recognising the need to advance from aid to mutual partnerships.

The need for wide coalitions to run major public health campaigns, was already recognised by the time of the polio initiative. From the beginning it was a broad coalition, led by WHO but with several partners. Rotary, as explained earlier, played a key role in both raising resources and persuading ministers and national health officials to take up the cause. Both the oncho and Guinea Worm campaigns are on a smaller scale. The 30 bilateral donors to the oncho programme, are organised by the World Bank. Merck's drug donation to the river blindness operation is organised by the independent Mectizan Donation Programme. The driving force behind Guinea Worm eradication has been the Carter Center.

LF is a much bigger programme. It requires a worldwide campaign. It needs WHO and a broad coalition of partners. That

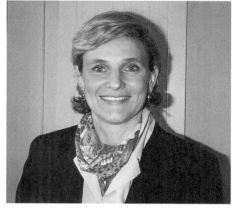

Maria Neira, Director, Eradication and Elimination, Communicable Diseases, WHO. She was a leader in helping Spain to host the first meeting of the Global Alliance in Santiago de Compostela.
Source: GSK

is what senior officials from WHO and GSK set out to create in 1998. Over at WHO, this was initially driven by Dr. Kazem Behbehani, the director of CTD (the control of tropical disease division) who played a key role in bringing on board the Arab Fund. After the 1998 restructuring, Dr. David Heymann, appointed executive director of the new communicable disease cluster, was in the driving seat assisted by Dr. Maria Neira, director of the department of control, prevention and eradication within the cluster.

Over at GSK, the key players were Brian Bagnall, director of GSK's LF project, and Doug Bauer, director of GSK's community partnership programme. At the suggestion of the two GSK players, a firm of interactive management consultants was commissioned to help prepare the ground for a partners' forum in Geneva at the end of October, 1998. People who doubt there was a need for an alliance, should look at the results of the survey carried out among potential partners and key public health figures before the forum met. Asked to identify objectives for the planned LF Global Alliance, the survey came up with 28 different goals. These included helping to shape the programme's vision; building a network of partners that could avoid turf wars through clearer understanding of partners' positions; mobilising wider international support for the programme while at the same time setting goals for creating community awareness and community involvement at the grass roots level. There was recognition that the Alliance would need to widen its focus from the many scientific and technical issues being explored, to the more mundane but equally important practical logistic concerns of managing a mass drug administration programme. Indeed, experienced hands saw the Alliance as an important vehicle for "sharing an understanding of the magnitude of the problems".

Other practical roles for the Alliance identified in the survey included participating in designing the programme's guidelines; exchanging technical information; identifying gaps in knowledge about the disease or the campaign and suggesting ways these could be filled; promoting co-ordination between partners; designing guidelines for morbidity control; and helping to integrate the many separate parts of an eradication programme—mapping, drug distribution, treatment, programme management and research. Wider roles ranged from "a reality check against inflated expectations for success" to "nurturing passionate support for the LF elimination programme". The list did not stop there but included "nurturing a belief in global health care philanthropy" and "looking beyond regionalism to global planning".

One measure of the progress achieved by the campaign is to look at the concerns raised at the partners' forum in Geneva in October, 1988, and to note the large number that had been resolved by the first meeting of the LF Global Alliance in Santiago 18 months later in May, 2000. In the survey carried out by the consultants before the Geneva conference, 28 technical barriers to global elimination were listed. This list was expanded by the 72 representatives from 30 organisations at the three-day conference to 51. They ranged across the spectrum. Some fundamental problems remain unresolved and are

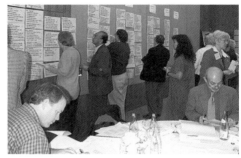

LF Partners' Forum, Geneva, October 1998.
Source: GSK

much bigger than LF: lack of health care finance; undertrained and over-worked health workers; the lack of a health care infrastructure in many countries.

The inadequate reach of many ministries of health was taken up in the pre-conference discussion paper. In many countries NGDOs (non-government development organisations) are delivering 60 per cent of health care services in rural areas. Delegates noted the conclusions of a report from a 1997 WHO study group (Regional Matters: reports by regional directors, technical report No 861) which itemised four particular health problems in developing countries: "lack of national health policies, fragmented health systems, limited resources, and poor management of available resources". In some countries these were exacerbated by weak

democratic structures and inadequate political commitment to
health. In some others there was concern that "an image of per-
vasive corruption within some ministries of health could have a
devastating impact". There was recognition that some countries
would not only need help in running a campaign (logistic support, inventory tracking, drug distribution) but also in preparing
applications.

These doubts contributed to a deep division on one issue
among those consulted: should states be required to draw up a
national LF elimination plan? Opponents believed NGDOs,
operating without the bureaucratic structures of many government organisations, had much more flexibility to set up new
models, that could then be replicated at the national level. They
expressed concern that NGDOs could lose operational impact if
they had to work through the ministry of health offices. Local
successful NGDO pilots could have the added advantage of raising the priority of the LF elimination programme within national
governments. They warned that "if care is not taken, the programme will end up treating too many people, too many times,
for too many years". The NGDO representatives wanted to "start
now" at the local level, so significant successes could be achieved
long before the ministries of health were able to complete the
development of their national plans and the Alliance's vetting
procedure approve them.

They lost the argument. For good reasons. Eradication campaigns require the full-hearted political backing of governments.
Without their active involvement, an eradication programme is
doomed. Ironically, during the smallpox campaign, there was little attempt by politicians to identify with the campaign, but in
subsequent public health operations—polio, roll back malaria,
Guinea Worm, river blindness—political leaders have learned the
degree to which such campaigns can help rally public support for
their governments.

Governments within developing countries do face harsh con-
flicting priorities. There is a problem of over-loading their
already over-loaded and frail health systems. In many countries

LF was not a high priority. But these problems cannot be resolved by ignoring them. The LF campaign is offering countries free drugs, which will not only help eliminate LF but also drastically reduce the prevalence of intestinal worms, scabies and lice. Eradication programmes can, as explained earlier, help to strengthen health systems. Delegates to the Geneva conference recognised there were all manner of other health programmes with which the LF campaign could be aligned. It was clear that a national plan did not imply that countries should launch nationwide. Pilots would be an important means of indicating the adjustments that might be needed to meet variable local conditions. Many would then only be able to to move to a phased introduction.

NGDOs, as subsequently demonstrated by the Carter Center's Global 2000 operation in Nigeria (See Chapter Five), could remain at the forefront of testing and supporting a national campaign. But there had to be a national plan which covered the wide range of operations in an eradication programme: mapping the disease to determine the extent of the treatment and drugs needed, working out drug distribution systems, training community health workers, monitoring reactions, mobilising funds, setting clear goals and most important of all, maintaining political commitment.

Many of the other doubts raised by delegates before Geneva are resolved. LF has a much higher profile—internationally and nationally—than two years ago. There has been no shortage of states applying to enrol in the campaign. By December 2000, over 40 of the 80 LF endemic states were already involved in the campaign: twelve had begun dual drug programmes; eleven had been given the go-ahead; seven were proceeding through the application process; three had completed action plans; and eight more had signalled an interest in enrolling in the programme.

Appropriately, Egypt, with perhaps the longest links with the disease—at least 4,000 years—was one of the first states to initiate a national programme under the Alliance. About 150,000 people, mostly in the eastern Nile delta, are infected and two million are at risk. Pilot programmes in two villages in early 2000

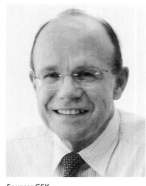

Source: GSK

BRIAN BAGNALL
A Missionary in Market Clothing

Beneath the private sector drive seeking efficiency and effectiveness, a missionary with zeal lives inside Brian Bagnall. As GSK's LF programme director, he is every bit as committed to helping the poor people who will benefit from the LF Global Alliance's campaign as the public health workers within the Alliance. They are the first to concede as much. It surfaced time and again in our interviews over three years.

He was an ideal scientist to take the lead LF role at GSK for two reasons: first, because of his early association with parasites, dermatology and albendazole—all key ingredients in the LF campaign. Second, given his various managerial positions including six years as vice president of government and industry affairs, he had already learned how to negotiate with governments and regulators. Setting up a global alliance requires interminable negotiations and consultations with public agencies.

Initially he trained as a vet in his native city, Sydney, Australia. Between his two post graduate degrees—also earned in Sydney—he joined Cambridge University's veterinary school as a clinician in the animal hospital, treating cases watched by an audience of students. Close scrutiny of his work holds no fear. While there he was awarded an Austrian government fellowship to spend a year at the University of Vienna studying veterinary dermatopathology. His Ph. D. in Sydney was in immunoparasitology, an appropriate background for a subsequent tropical disease eradicator.

Returning to the U.K. after his doctorate, his first project with GSK, as technical services officer, was steering albendazole through its licensing hoops. Like most anti-worm pills, it was originally launched for use with animals, first being introduced in New Zealand/Australia for sheep in 1977. Brian negotiated U.K. regulatory approval the following year. Ironically, after its early success, the drug was overtaken by ivermectin because Merck had designed a method of injecting its drug, rather than requiring that pills be put down animal throats.

He worked in GSK's animal health division holding a variety of scientific and managerial positions for 18 years. The public health agencies pay tribute to the speed and flexibility with which GSK is able to reach decisions and act. There is no bureaucracy in the LF unit. Brian Bagnall is used to making decisions.

One of his great strengths is the ability to recognise the pressure under which other organisations are working—a key skill in putting together an alliance. He is a shrewd reader of other people's problems. At an early meeting of GSK officials, I watched senior company officials worry whether Merck would join the LF Global Alliance. Bagnall remained calm, unperturbed and confident that they would. He read their position extremely accurately. They had been funding the river blindness campaign for 12 years. Other contributors to that campaign were beginning to get donor fatigue. Bagnall summed it up with insight and accuracy: "Of course they should be careful, with regulatory rules, but they will collaborate because they have a humanitarian heart."

His Australian accent gives him an advantage. He always sounds laid back, but beneath that relaxed exterior is a fierce drive. He'd make an excellent journalist. I followed some of his trails—to Haiti and Brazil—three months behind him. His reports were always succinctly written and provided an invaluable and vivid map to those in his wake.

What's his new job like? "Much harder work than I imagined. In some stormy squalls I thought I would go mad. When you create a public/private alliance of this size and complexity, it is not easy. There are lots of meetings, talks, debates and disagreements. The Gates money could have broken the Alliance, when it asked the separate parties to work out how to spend it, but instead it cemented us."

"Above all, the job has been a humbling experience. I have had the privilege of working with some of the finest humanitarian scientists and academics in world medicine. And I've been inspired even more by the LF patients I have met. Once you go on a field trip and see the progress that is being made, administrative headaches fall into perspective." What have been the high points? "The Gates cash; the Partners' Forum in Geneva in 1998 when it became clear the key partners were climbing aboard; the first formal meeting of the LF Global Alliance in Spain in 2000."

What lessons has he learned? "You need vision and you have to take risks. Tropical diseases are so well entrenched and widespread, they need a response of equal size. Global alliances are the only way forward. Hopefully, in another decade's time, company donations like GSK's LF commitment will no longer be seen as novel."

achieved remarkable success covering 96% of the eligible population. The main programme was launched in the third quarter, based on house-to-house visits by pairs of community health workers, to ensure that each family member took the LF medication. Alliance observers returned full of enthusiasm for the political commitment that was invested in the Egyptian campaign. It was led by a dynamic head of communicable diseases in WHO's Eastern Mediterranean Region, who pushed and prodded a wide cross-section of supporters. Launched in an election year, it won the unequivocal support of political leaders, who backed a national plan of almost military detail, and ensured there was comprehensive coverage in the local media. Large numbers of physicians and nurses were recruited to back up the local teams. Of the 1.8 million targeted in 2000, some 1.75 million were treated.

In other parts of the world, the South Pacific is steaming ahead (See Chapter Four). Four African states began programmes in 2000. Tanzania treated 23,000 people and Nigeria 160,000. Togo was targeting 77,000 people and Ghana 480,000. The 12 national programmes that were launched in 2000 reached 3.2 million people. With the launch of the Indian programme in 2001, with a pilot covering 20 million that eventually will need to widen and cover 450 million people, total treatment numbers are rising exponentially. The number of people treated is projected to rise to 40 million people in 27 countries during 2001.

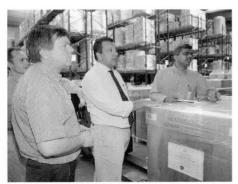

WHO visits the GSK albendazole manufacturing facility in Mayenne, France (L–R foreground: Steve Lyons, Nevio Zagaria and Gautam Biswas). Shipment box contains 480,000 tablets bound for Ghana.
Source: GSK

Other new programmes in 2001 include Bangladesh (1 million), Sri Lanka, Myanmar and Vietnam (all 2 million)

The widespread concern about what can be done to help the victims of the disease has begun to abate with the success of

Gerusa Dreyer's clinics in Brazil described to both the London and Spanish conferences (See Chapter Six). Similar clinics are springing up in other countries and international programmes for health trainers have already begun. Educational materials have been produced—for clinics and eradication campaigners. Even better, national campaigners have been encouraging their own people—patients, children, health workers—to produce their own material in their own language. These range from jingles for radio campaigns, songs for community meetings, through to poems, paintings and books for schools.

There are no longer any doubts from hard core sceptics about GSK's commitment to donate albendazole or Merck's readiness to supply ivermectin free of charge. SmithKline Beecham merged with Glaxo Wellcome in late 2000, but reassurance about the LF programme was one of the earliest commitments of the new company, GlaxoSmithKline. Like SB, Glaxo had its own philanthropic programme including a malaria drug donation programme. SB's LF campaign helped win for the company the 1998 Business Ethics Magazine award celebrating best practice in social responsibility. The $1 billion SB commitment was described as "unparalleled in scope". GSK has not confined its philanthropy to drug donations but backed up the campaign by helping to finance the succession of task forces, conferences, working groups and research initiatives that have been necessary to get the programme rolling. It is helping to finance the LF support centre at the Liverpool School of Tropical Medicine, funded cost/benefit studies at Emory University, Atlanta and is helping to finance Dr. Dreyer's drive to improve the health care of existing patients.

GSK and Merck worked out ways of coordinating their drug supplies to Africa. Concern over the safety of the dual drug programme, despite the millions who had taken the drugs separately, was assuaged by a rigorous re-examination of the dual drug trials. WHO collected copies of all the original data forms used to record safety observations of the trials. This material was gathered for further clinical safety analysis by Prof. Jens Schou (consultant to WHO) and GSK's Dr. John Horton. Further assessments were made by four medical members of WHO staff (Drs. Lazdins, Ottesen, Savioli and Couper) and Merck's Dr. Alfred Saah. Separate reports were produced on the separate combinations. The reviews recommended, and the programme accepted, a requirement that each new national programme begins with a pilot programme of 2,000 patients under which all effects are closely monitored and reported back to Geneva. The LF Alliance reports back at six- and 12-month intervals on national programmes for the first five years of the campaign. WHO has produced new procedures for ensuring a high quality supply of DEC to end the previous wide variations in standards, strength and price. It is also investigating the development of a chewable DEC tablet, following the success of the albendazole tablet manufactured for the campaign, which was sweetened to make it more attractive to children and does not need water to be swallowed, giving it an additional benefit in areas of contaminated water.

A draft strategic plan for the campaign was published in June, 1999, and a revised version in September 1999, complete with a timetable and specific goals for each of the next five years ending in 2004. The number of people covered was expected to rise from 20 million by the end of 2000 to 200 million by the end of 2004. By the end of 2001, the aim was to have completed mapping in more than half of endemic countries in all regions.

The aim of the first five year phase is to demonstrate success, confirm the treatment regime, clarify any safety features, test the mass drug administration logistics and implement an effective monitoring and assessment procedure. Three further phases follow. The first year has already demonstrated that mass drug administration is feasible, an LF programme can be integrated and help strengthen national health structures, and the potential for linking to other public health programmes (river blindness, schisto, malaria) looks exceedingly promising (See Chapter Five).

One major worry at the Geneva forum was over the authorisation procedure. Delegates expressed concern that it would be too top heavy if all applications had to be approved from a single centre in WHO's Geneva headquarters. The debate continued through 1999 and was finally resolved at a meeting of the major partners at the World Bank's offices in London in December 1999. It was agreed that the Programme Review Group (PRG) established by WHO in Geneva to vet national applications, would continue for up to a further two years to oversee the launch of the programme worldwide and ensure that momentum was maintained and increased. All governments applying to join the campaign were required to submit national plans of action, including detailed breakdowns of the drug donations that would be needed, to the PRG through WHO. Once full momentum has been achieved, the plan is to decentralise the PRG process to regional level.

The same December meeting agreed on two other constitutional issues. First, the Technical Advisory Group (TAG), a group of specialists selected for their personal expertise in LF science and programme management, is to meet annually to give their recommendations on all aspects of the elimination effort in all regions of the world. The aim will be to ensure that TAG members, selected in consultation with the programme's partners, will provide a balance of technical and regional representation. Allied campaigns—river blindness and malaria—would also be represented. One third of the members will change each year. Consecutive appointments will not normally occur. TAG meetings will be open to representatives of the LF partners to encourage open debate and give the widest opportunity for alternative views. As the regional programmes develop, regional TAGs will be encouraged to address the special needs of regions.

The second constitutional issue settled was the role of the Alliance. Membership is open to all interested parties. Its main purpose is to act as a forum for the exchange of ideas and co-ordination of activities. Its other functions include raising international awareness of LF; and attracting new partners. The Alliance will not normally meet more frequently than once a year. The second gathering is planned for India in early 2002, when the eradication programme in the subcontinent will already be in full swing.

Funding remains a concern. That was why the $20 million donation over five years from the Gates Foundation was such a fillip. Hopefully, there will be more from that source. Bill Foege has been recruited by Bill Gates to be his main health adviser. No one is more aware than Foege of the funding an eradication programme requires. The $20 million donation looks like a marker. It came at an early stage of the eradication campaign, when the LF Global Alliance was still proving itself. The early programmes, set out above, are providing the necessary proof. Eric Ottesen, at its heart, could not be more enthusiastic about the momentum that is being achieved. He talks of the exhilaration that the accelerating progress is generating. National aid agencies are backing the campaign—Australia, Belgium, Italy, Japan, the Netherlands, Spain and the U.K. Japan, for example, is funding much of the work across the Pacific. The Arab Fund for Economic and Social Development was one of the earliest funders, supporting programmes in the Middle East. The NDGOs are joining in and expanding the work on the ground (See list below). The two big drug companies have provided all manner of support as well as free drugs. Yet, as Anne Haddix has shown and I reported in Chapter One, big bucks are needed: an estimated $600 million in the first five years over and above the $400 million in free drug donations. Hesitant donors, please cough up more.

The first meeting of the LF Global Alliance in Spain in May 2000, demonstrated its inclusiveness and the high morale among campaigners, now that the programme was underway. Paul Derstine, president of Interchurch Medical Assistance and chair of the NGDO Co-ordination Group, said the Alliance was a means of ensuring the LF campaign maintained its three-pronged approach. He saw the Alliance as "a three legged stool", comprising public, private and non-profit partners. The Alliance would ensure the voice of the NGDOs would be heard. Until its creation, the road had been "littered with unclear road signs". One important way all parties were involved was in the six separate workshops at the conference that covered a broad sweep of issues. These included information needs, funding, the role of NGDOs in supporting national programmes, the role of the Alliance in supporting national campaigns, and maximising regional coordination. Phil Mason, head of the health and population division of the U.K.'s Department for International Development (DFID) which helped finance the conference, noted the enormous progress that had been achieved since Geneva and suggested: "Great ideas need landing gear as well as wings. This inaugural meeting of the Alliance has shown the wings are in good order— and the landing gear is now being defined with the help from the working groups." He added: "When the history of this programme comes to be written, this meeting may be seen as the real starting point for actually getting down to business."

Dr. Bernhard Liese, the World Bank's senior adviser on human development in the African region, warned the conference that there was still a long hill to climb requiring "stamina, strength and endurance". It would be important to walk on two legs—tackling both the interruption of transmission and disability control. On the first front, substantial progress had been achieved in a short period of time, especially through the safety of drug combinations; but on the second, a lot of work remained to be done. Summing up, he declared: "The first big step has been made. The LF Global Alliance has moved from infancy to being a toddler—one with many parents, all of whom share a commitment to a common cause: placing the elimination of LF higher on the world's development agenda and to restoring dignity, respect and health to its victims."

The full membership of the Alliance comprises:

National Ministries of Health
- Ministries of Health of *endemic countries*

International Organizations
- The World Bank
- United Nations Children's Fund—UNICEF
- World Health Organization—WHO

Private Sector
- Binax, Inc., United States of America
- Merck & Co., Inc., United States of America
- GlaxoSmithKline, United Kingdom

International Development Agencies
- Arab Fund for Social and Economic Development (AFSED), Kuwait
- Centers for Disease Control and Prevention (CDC), Atlanta, United States of America
- Department for International Development (DFID), United Kingdom
- Directorate General for Development Cooperation (DGCS), Italy
- Japan International Cooperation Agency (JICA), Japan
- Ministry of Health and Welfare, Japan
- Ministère fédéral des Affaires sociales, de la Santé publique et de l'Environnment, Belgium
- Ministerio de Sanidad Y Consumo, Spain
- Ministry of Health Welfare and Sport, Netherlands
- Vector Control Research Centre (VCRC), Indian Council of Medical Research, India

Non-Governmental Organizations
- Amaury Couthino, Brazil
- The Carter Center, USA
- Centres for Partnerships in Health, Australia
- Handicap International, France
- Health and Development International (HDI), Norway
- Interchurch Medical Assistance (IMA), United States of America
- International Volunteers in Urology, United States of America
- Mectizan® Donation Program, United States of America
- World Alliance for Community Health, Canada

Academia

- Ain Shams University, Egypt
- Bernhard Nocht Institute for Tropical Medicine, Germany
- Chinese Academy of Preventive Medicine, China
- Danish Bilharziasis Laboratory (DBL), Denmark
- Emory University, Atlanta, United States of America
- Institute for Medical Research (IMR), Malaysia
- James Cook University, Australia
- Liverpool School of Tropical Medicine—LF Support Centre, United Kingdom
- Michigan State University, United States of America
- Notre Dame University, United States of America
- Universidade Federal de Pernambuco, Brazil
- Washington University in St. Louis—Barnes-Jewish Hospital, United States of America